Surgery at a Glance

Surgery at a Glance

Pierce A. Grace

MCh, FRCSI, FRCS
Professor of Surgical Science
University of Limerick
Midwestern Regional Hospital
Limerick

Neil R. Borley

FRCS, FRCS (Ed) MS
Consultant Colorectal Surgeon
Cheltenham General Hospital
Cheltenham

Third edition

Blackwell
Publishing

First published 1999
Second edition 2002
Reprinted 2003, 2004, 2005
Third edition 2006

Library of Congress Cataloging-in-Publication Data

Grace, P. A. (Pierce A.)
    Surgery at a glance / Pierce A. Grace, Neil R. Borley. – 3rd ed.
        p. ; cm.
    Includes index.
    ISBN-13: 978-1-4051-3187-2 (alk. paper)
    ISBN-10: 1-4051-3187-X (alk. paper)
    1. Diagnosis, Surgical–Handbooks, manuals, etc.   2. Operations,
Surgical–Handbooks, manuals, etc.   3. Surgery–Handbooks, manuals,
etc.   I. Borley, Neil R.   II. Title.
    [DNLM: 1. Surgical Procedures, Operative–Handbooks.   2. Diagnosis–
Handbooks.   WO 39 G729c 2006]
    RD35.G68 2006
    617′.9–dc22   2005017901

ISBN-13: 978-1-4051-3187-2
ISBN-10: 1-4051-3187-X

A catalogue record for this title is available from the British Library

Set in 9.5/12pt Times by Graphicraft Limited, Hong Kong
Printed and bound in India by Replika Press Pvt. Ltd

Commissioning Editor: Vicki Noyes
Development Editor: Karen Moore
Production Controller: Kate Charman

For further information on Blackwell Publishing, visit our website: http://www.blackwellpublishing.com

The publisher's policy is to use permanent paper from mills that operate a sustainable forestry policy, and
which has been manufactured from pulp processed using acid-free and elementary chlorine-free practices.
Furthermore, the publisher ensures that the text paper and cover board used have met acceptable
environmental accreditation standards.

Contents

Preface

We are very pleased to present the third edition of *Surgery at a Glance*. This book is now a firm favourite with medical students internationally for learning and revising undergraduate surgery for the final MB examination. Others, who require an overview of clinical surgery, for example, nursing students and postgraduate surgical students, also find *Surgery at a Glance* a very helpful text.

This new edition follows the same format as the previous editions but some significant changes have been made. Firstly, more colour has been used in the production of the new edition and we feel that this gives the book a very bright and user-friendly look. The 'Key Points' and 'Key Investigations' sections of the text are more easily read and the use of colour has transformed the illustrations. Secondly, five new chapters (Anaesthesia, Surgical Infections, Lymphoedema, Incisions & Stomas, and Solid Organ Transplantation) have been added and the rest of the book has been revised to acknowledge the constant evolution of surgical practice. The overall appearance and structure of the book remains the same. Each chapter is presented across a two-page spread, illustrations on the left-hand page and text on the right. Part 1 (Clinical Presentations at a Glance, 28 chapters) concentrates on the symptoms and signs with which patients present, while Part 2 (Surgical Diseases at a Glance, 55 chapters) is concerned with the common surgical diseases. The revisions to the third edition have been achieved without a major increase in size of the book.

We have had much help from several people in putting this book together. We would like to thank the many medical students and colleagues who have read the book and given us good suggestions. We would especially like to thank the team at Blackwell Publishing including Fiona Goodgame, Karen Moore, Geraldine Jeffers and Mirjana Misina for their encouragement, patience and professionalism in bringing the project to fruition. We thank the illustrators especially for their excellent illustrations.

We believe that the third edition of *Surgery at a Glance* is a very modern surgical text that will help the student understand how patients present with 'surgical' problems and how they might be managed. We hope you will enjoy it and learn from it.

Pierce Grace
Neil Borley
2005

List of Abbreviations

AAA	abdominal aortic aneurysm		**DU**	duodenal ulcer
AAT	aspartate amino transferase		**DVT**	deep venous thrombosis
ABI	ankle–brachial pressure index		**Dx**	diagnosis
Ach	acetylcholine		**DXT**	deep X-ray therapy
ACN	acute cortical necrosis		**EAS**	external anal sphincter
ACTH	adrenocorticotrophic hormone		**EBV**	Epstein–Barr virus
ADH	antidiuretic hormone		**ECG**	electrocardiogram
Adr	adrenaline/epinephrine		**ER**	oestrogen receptor
AF	atrial fibrillation		**ERCP**	endoscopic retrograde cholangiopancreatographic (examination)
AFP	α-fetoprotein			
Ag	antigen		**ESR**	erythrocyte sedimentation rate
Alb	albumin		**ESWL**	extracorporeal shock-wave lithotripsy
ANCA	anti-neutrophil cytoplasmic antibody		**EUA**	examination under anaesthesia
ANDI	abnormalities of the normal development and involution (of the breast)		**FBC**	full blood count
			FCD	fibrocystic disease
AP	anteroposterior		**FHx**	family history
APTT	activated partial thromboplastin time		**FNAC**	fine-needle aspiration cytology
ARDS	adult/acute respiratory distress syndrome		**FOB**	faecal occult blood
ARF	acute renal failure		**FSH**	follicle-stimulating hormone
ATN	acute tubular necrosis		**5-FU**	5-fluorouracil
AVM	arteriovenous malfunction		**γ-GT**	gamma glutamyl transpeptidase
AXR	abdominal X-ray		**GA**	general anaesthetic
BCC	basal cell carcinoma		**GCS**	Glasgow Coma Scale
BCG	bacillus Calmette–Guérin		**GFR**	glomerular filtration rate
BE	base excess		**GH**	growth hormone
BP	blood pressure		**GI**	gastrointestinal
BPH	benign prostatic hypertrophy		**GORD**	gastro-oesophageal reflux disease
C&S	culture and sensitivity		**GTN**	glyceryl trinitrate
CABG	coronary artery bypass graft		**GU**	genito-urinary
CBD	common bile duct		**Hb**	haemoglobin
CCF	congestive cardiac failure		**β-HCG**	β-human chorionic gonadotrophin
CD	*Clostridium difficile*		**HCG**	human chorionic gonadotrophin
CEA	carcinoembryonic antigen		**Hct**	haematocrit
CK	creatinine kinase		**HDU**	high-dependency unit
CLO	*Campylobacter*-like organism		**HIDA**	imido-diacetic acid
CMV	cytomegalovirus		**HLA**	human leucocyte antigen
CNS	central nervous system		**Hx**	history
COCP	combined oral contraceptive pill		**IBS**	irritable bowel syndrome
COPD	chronic obstructive pulmonary disease		**ICP**	intracranial pressure
CPK-MB	creatine phosphokinase (cardiac type)		**ICS**	intercostal space
CRC	colorectal carcinoma		**ICU**	intensive care unit
CRF	chronic renal failure		**IgG**	immunoglobulin G
CRP	C-reactive protein		**IPPV**	intermittent positive pressure ventilation
CSF	cerebrospinal fluid		**ITP**	idiopathic thrombocytopaenic purpura
CT	computed tomography		**IVC**	inferior vena cava
CVA	cerebrovascular accident		**IVU**	intravenous urogram
CVP	central venous pressure		**JGA**	juxtaglomerular apparatus
CXR	chest X-ray		**JVP**	jugular venous pulse
D$_2$	type 2 dopaminergic receptors		**LA**	local anaesthetic
DIC	disseminated intravascular coagulation		**LAD**	left anterior descending
DMSA	dimercaptosuccinic acid		**LATS**	long-acting thyroid stimulating (factor)
Dop	dopamine		**LCA**	left coronary artery
DPTA	diethylenetriaminepentaacetic acid		**LDH**	lactate dehydrogenase

LFT	liver function test	**PT**	prothrombin time
LH	luteinizing hormone	**PTC**	percutaneous transhepatic cholangiography
LH-RH	LH-releasing hormone	**PTH**	parathyroid hormone
LIF	left iliac fossa	**PUD**	peptic ulcer disease
LOC	loss of consciousness	**PUO**	pyrexia of unknown origin
LOS	lower oesophageal sphincter	**PV**	per vaginum
LPS	lipopolysaccharide	**PVD**	peripheral vascular disease
LSE	left sternal edge	**RBC**	red blood cell
LSF	lesser sciatica foramen	**RCC**	renal cell carcinoma
LUQ	left upper quadrant	**RIA**	radioimmunoassay
LV	left ventricle	**RIF**	right iliac fossa
LVF	left ventricular failure	**RLN**	recurrent laryngeal nerve
MC+S	microscopy cultures and sensitivity	**RPLND**	retroperitoneal lymph node dissection
MCP	metacarpophalangeal	**RT**	radiotherapy
MEN	multiple endocrine neoplasia	**RUQ**	right upper quadrant
MI	myocardial infarction	**RV**	right ventricle
MIBG	*meta*-iodo-benzyl guanidine	**RVF**	right ventricular failure
MM	malignant melanoma	**Rx**	treatment
MND	motor neurone disease	**SCC**	squamous cell carcinoma
MODS	multiple organ dysfunction syndrome	**SFJ**	sapheno-femoral junction
MRA	magnetic resonance angiography	**SGOT**	serum glutamic oxalacetic transaminase
MRCP	magnetic resonance cholangio-pancreatography	**SIADH**	syndrome of inappropriate antidiuretic hormone
MRI	magnetic resonance imaging	**SIRS**	systemic inflammatory response syndrome
MS	multiple sclerosis	**SLE**	systemic lupus erythematosus
MSH	melanocyte-stimulating hormone	**SLN**	superior laryngeal nerve
MSU	mid-stream urine	**STD**	sodium tetradecyl
MT	major trauma	**SVC**	superior vena cava
MTP	metatarsophalangeal	**Sxr**	skull X-ray
MUGA	multiple uptake gated analysis	**T₃**	T_3 tri-iodothyronine
NAdr	noradrenaline/norepinephrine	**T₄**	T_4 thyroxine
NG	nasogastric	**TB**	tuberculosis
NSAID	non-steroidal anti-inflammatory drug	**TCC**	transitional cell carcinoma
NSU	non-specific urethritis	**TED**	thrombo-embolic deterrent
OA	osteoarthritis	**TIA**	transient ischaemic attack
OGD	oesophago-gastro-duodenoscopy	**TNM**	tumour, node, metastasis (UICC)
OGJ	oesophago-gastric junction	**t-PA**	tissue plasminogen activator
PA	posteroanterior	**TPHA**	treponema pallidum haemagglutination (test)
PAF	platelet activating factor	**TPR**	temperature, pulse, respiration
PCA	patient-controlled analgesia	**TSH**	thyroid-stimulating hormone
PCV	packed cell volume	**TURP**	transurethral resection of the prostate
PE	pulmonary embolism	**TURT**	transurethral resection of tumour
PHx	past history	**UC**	ulcerative colitis
PID	pelvic inflammatory disease	**UDT**	undescended testis
PIP	proximal interphalangeal	**U+E**	urea and electrolytes
PL	prolactin	**UTI**	urinary tract infection
PMN	polymorphonuclear leucocyte	**VA**	visual acuity
POVD	peripheral occlusive vascular disease	**VHL**	von Hippel–Lindau
PPI	proton pump inhibitor	**VIP**	vasoactive intestinal peptide
PPL	postphlebitic limb	**VMA**	vanillyl mandelic acid
PR	per rectum	**VSD**	ventricular septal defect
PSA	prostate-specific antigen	**WCC**	white cell count

1 Neck lump

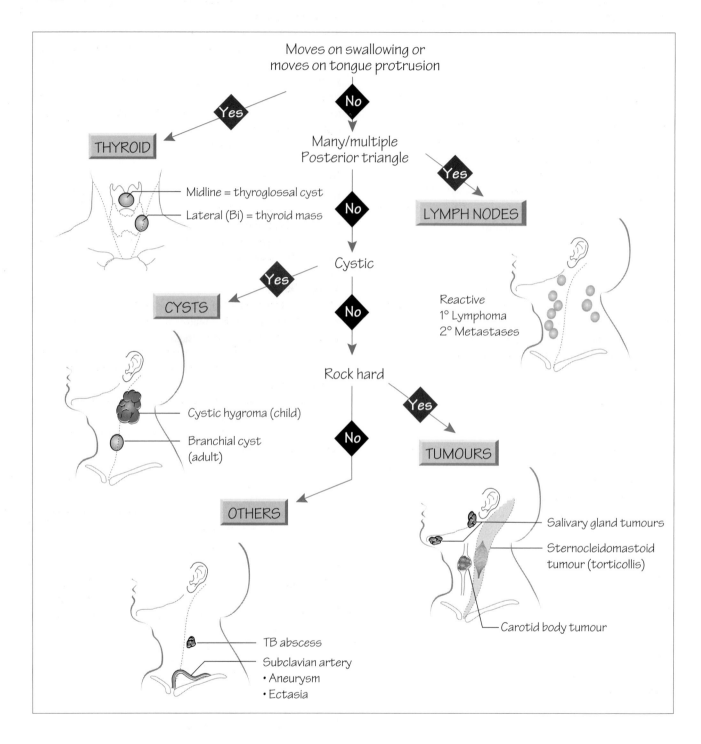

Moves on swallowing or
moves on tongue protrusion

No → Many/multiple
Posterior triangle

Yes → THYROID

Midline = thyroglossal cyst
Lateral (Bi) = thyroid mass

Yes → LYMPH NODES

Reactive
1° Lymphoma
2° Metastases

No → Cystic

Yes → CYSTS

Cystic hygroma (child)
Branchial cyst (adult)

No → Rock hard

Yes → TUMOURS

Salivary gland tumours
Sternocleidomastoid tumour (torticollis)
Carotid body tumour

No → OTHERS

TB abscess
Subclavian artery
• Aneurysm
• Ectasia

Definition

A *neck lump* is any congenital or acquired mass arising in the anterior or posterior triangles of the neck between the clavicles inferiorly and the mandible and base of the skull superiorly.

Key points

- Thyroid swellings move upwards (with the trachea) on swallowing.
- Most abnormalities of the neck are visible as swellings.
- Ventral lumps attached to the hyoid bone, such as thyroglossal cysts, move upwards with both swallowing and protrusion of the tongue.
- Multiple lumps are almost always lymph nodes.
- Don't forget a full head and neck examination, including the oral cavity, in all cases of lymphadenopathy.

Differential diagnosis

- 50% of neck lumps are thyroid in origin.
- 40% of neck lumps are caused by malignancy (80% metastatic usually from primary lesion above the clavicle; 20% primary neoplasms: lymphomas, salivary gland tumours).
- 10% of neck lumps are inflammatory or congenital in origin.

Thyroid

- Goitre, cyst, neoplasm.

Neoplasm

- Metastatic carcinoma.
- Primary lymphoma.
- Salivary gland tumour.
- Sternocleidomastoid tumour.
- Carotid body tumour.

Inflammatory

- Acute infective adenopathy.
- Collar stud abscess.
- Cystic hygroma.
- Branchial cyst.
- Parotitis.

Congenital

- Thyroglossal duct cyst.
- Dermoid cyst.
- Torticollis.

Vascular

- Subclavian aneurysm.
- Subclavian ectasia.

Important diagnostic features

Children

Congenital and inflammatory lesions are common.

- Cystic hygroma: in infants, base of the neck, brilliant transillumination, 'come and go'.
- Thyroglossal or dermoid cyst: midline, discrete, elevates with tongue protrusion.
- Torticollis: rock-hard mass, more prominent with head flexed, associated with fixed rotation (a fibrous mass in the sternocleidomastoid muscle).
- Branchial cyst: anterior to the upper third of the sternocleidomastoid.
- Viral/bacterial adenitis: usually affects jugular nodes, multiple, tender masses.
- Neoplasms are unusual in children (lymphoma most common).

Young adults

Inflammatory neck masses and thyroid malignancy are common.

- Viral (e.g. infectious mononucleosis) or bacterial (tonsillitis/pharyngitis) adenitis.
- Papillary thyroid cancer: isolated, non-tender, thyroid mass, possible lymphadenopathy.

Over-40s

Neck lumps are malignant until proven otherwise.

- Metastatic lymphadenopathy: multiple, rock-hard, non-tender, tendency to be fixed.
- 75% in primary head and neck (thyroid, nasopharynx, tonsils, larynx, pharynx), 25% from infraclavicular primary (stomach, pancreas, lung).
- Primary lymphadenopathy (thyroid, lymphoma): fleshy, matted, rubbery, large size.
- Primary neoplasm (thyroid, salivary tumour): firm, non-tender, fixed to tissue of origin.

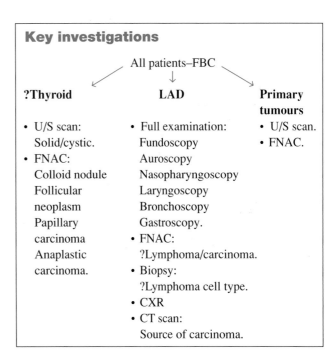

Key investigations

All patients–FBC

?Thyroid | **LAD** | **Primary tumours**

?Thyroid
- U/S scan: Solid/cystic.
- FNAC: Colloid nodule Follicular neoplasm Papillary carcinoma Anaplastic carcinoma.

LAD
- Full examination: Fundoscopy Auroscopy Nasopharyngoscopy Laryngoscopy Bronchoscopy Gastroscopy.
- FNAC: ?Lymphoma/carcinoma.
- Biopsy: ?Lymphoma cell type.
- CXR
- CT scan: Source of carcinoma.

Primary tumours
- U/S scan.
- FNAC.

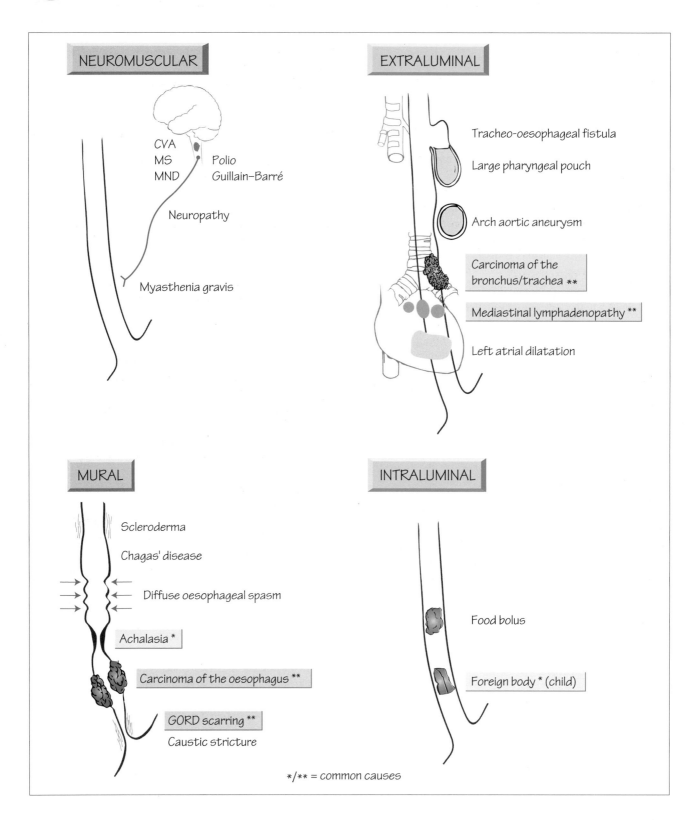

NEUROMUSCULAR

CVA
MS   Polio
MND   Guillain–Barré

Neuropathy

Myasthenia gravis

EXTRALUMINAL

Tracheo-oesophageal fistula

Large pharyngeal pouch

Arch aortic aneurysm

Carcinoma of the
bronchus/trachea **

Mediastinal lymphadenopathy **

Left atrial dilatation

MURAL

Scleroderma

Chagas' disease

Diffuse oesophageal spasm

Achalasia *

Carcinoma of the oesophagus **

GORD scarring **

Caustic stricture

INTRALUMINAL

Food bolus

Foreign body * (child)

*/** = common causes

Definition

Dysphagia literally means difficulty with swallowing, which may be associated with ingestion of solids or liquids or both.

Key points

- Most causes of dysphagia are oesophageal in origin.
- In children, foreign bodies and corrosive liquids are common causes.
- In young adults, reflux stricture and achalasia are common.
- In the middle aged and elderly, carcinoma and reflux are common.
- Because the segmental nerve supply of the oesophagus corresponds to the intercostal dermatomes, a patient with dysphagia can accurately pinpoint the level of obstruction.
- Any new symptoms of progressive dysphagia should be assumed to be malignant until proven otherwise. All need endoscopic or radiological investigation.
- Tumour and achalasia may mimic each other. Endoscopy and biopsy are advisable unless the diagnosis is clear.

Important diagnostic features
Mural

- Carcinoma of the oesophagus: progressive course, associated weight loss and anorexia, low-grade anaemia, possible small haematemesis.
- Reflux oesophagitis and stricture: preceded by heartburn, progressive course, nocturnal regurgitation.
- Achalasia: onset in young adulthood or old age, liquids disproportionately difficult to swallow, frequent regurgitation, recurrent chest infections, long history.
- Tracheo-oesophageal fistula: recurrent chest infections, coughing after drinking. Present in childhood (congenital) or late adulthood (post trauma, deep X-ray therapy (DXT) or malignant).
- Chagas' disease (*Trypanosoma cruzi*): South American prevalence, associated with dysrhythmias and colonic dysmotility.

- Caustic stricture: examination shows corrosive ingestion, chronic dysphagia, onset may be months after.
- Scleroderma: slow onset, associated with skin and hair changes.

Intraluminal

Foreign body: acute onset, marked retrosternal discomfort, dysphagia even to saliva is characteristic.

Extramural

- Pulsion diverticulum: intermittent symptoms, unexpected regurgitation.
- External compression: mediastinal lymph nodes, left atrial hypertrophy, bronchial malignancy.

Key investigations

All
FBC: anaemia (tumours much more commonly cause this than reflux).
LFTs: (hepatic disease).
↓
OGD
(moderate risk, specialist, good for differentiating tumour vs. achalasia vs. reflux stricture, allows biopsy for tissue diagnosis, allows possible treatment).
Barium swallow
(low risk, easy, good for possible fistula, high tumour, diverticulum, reflux).
↓

If ?dysmotility	If ?extrinsic compression
- achalasia	↓
- neurogenic causes	CXR (AP and lateral)
↓	CT scan: low risk, good
Video barium swallow	for extrinsic compression,
Oesophageal manometry	allows tumour staging

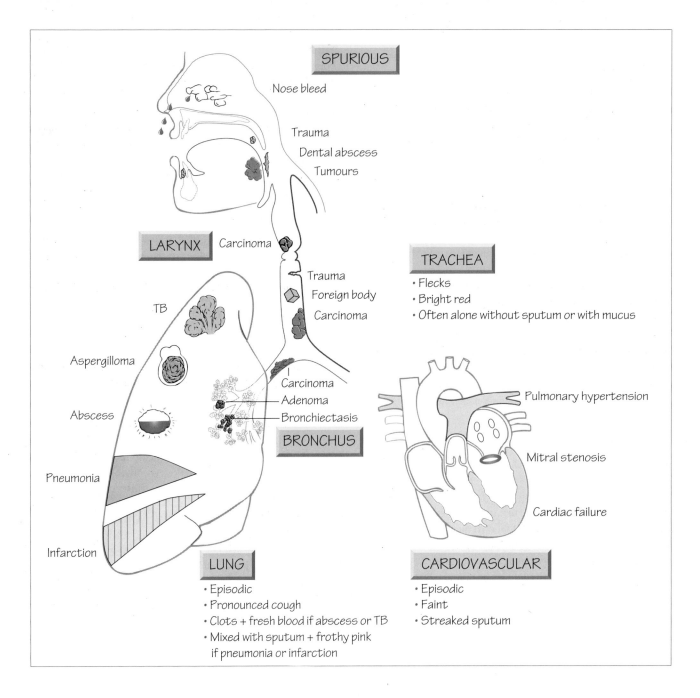

SPURIOUS

Nose bleed

Trauma

Dental abscess

Tumours

LARYNX

Carcinoma

TRACHEA
- Flecks
- Bright red
- Often alone without sputum or with mucus

Trauma

Foreign body

Carcinoma

TB

Aspergilloma

Carcinoma
Adenoma
Bronchiectasis

BRONCHUS

Abscess

Pulmonary hypertension

Mitral stenosis

Cardiac failure

Pneumonia

Infarction

LUNG
- Episodic
- Pronounced cough
- Clots + fresh blood if abscess or TB
- Mixed with sputum + frothy pink
  if pneumonia or infarction

CARDIOVASCULAR
- Episodic
- Faint
- Streaked sputum

Definition

Haemoptysis (blood spitting) is the symptom of coughing up blood from the lungs. Blood from the nose, mouth or pharynx that may also be spat out is termed 'spurious haemoptysis'.

Key points

- Blood from the proximal bronchi or trachea is usually bright red. It may be frankly blood or mixed with mucus and debris, particularly from a tumour.
- Blood from the distal bronchioles and alveoli is often pink and mixed with frothy sputum.

Important diagnostic features

The sources, causes and features are listed below.

Spurious haemoptysis

Mouth and nose

- Blood dyscrasias: associated nose bleeds, spontaneous bruising.
- Scurvy (vitamin C deficiency): poor hair/teeth, skin bruising.
- Dental caries, trauma, gingivitis.
- Oral tumours: painful intraoral mass, discharge, fetor.
- Hypertensive/spontaneous: no warning, brief bleed, often recurrent.
- Nasal tumours (common in South-East Asia).

True haemoptysis

Larynx and trachea

- Foreign body: choking, stridor, pain.
- Carcinoma: hoarse voice, bovine cough.

Bronchus

- Carcinoma: spontaneous haemoptysis, chest infections, weight loss, monophonic wheezing.
- Adenoma (e.g. carcinoid): recurrent chest infections, carcinoid syndrome.
- Bronchiectasis: chronic chest infections, fetor, blood mixed with purulent sputum, physical examination shows TB or severe chest infections.
- Foreign body: recurrent chest infections, sudden-onset inexplicable 'asthma'.

Lung

- TB: weight loss, fevers, night sweats, dry or productive cough.
- Pneumonia/lung abscess: features of acute chest sepsis, swinging fever.
- Pulmonary infarct (secondary to PE): pleuritic chest pain, tachypnoea, pleural rub.
- Aspergilloma.

Cardiac

- Mitral stenosis: frothy pink sputum, recurrent chest infections.
- LVF: frothy pink sputum, pulmonary oedema.

Key investigations

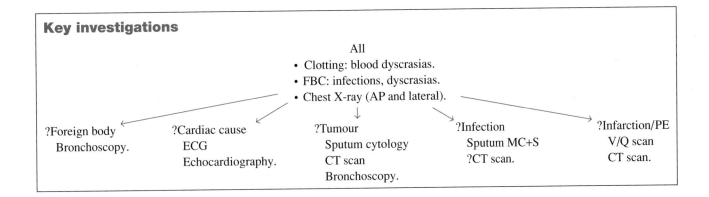

All
- Clotting: blood dyscrasias.
- FBC: infections, dyscrasias.
- Chest X-ray (AP and lateral).

?Foreign body
Bronchoscopy.

?Cardiac cause
ECG
Echocardiography.

?Tumour
Sputum cytology
CT scan
Bronchoscopy.

?Infection
Sputum MC+S
?CT scan.

?Infarction/PE
V/Q scan
CT scan.

4 Breast lump

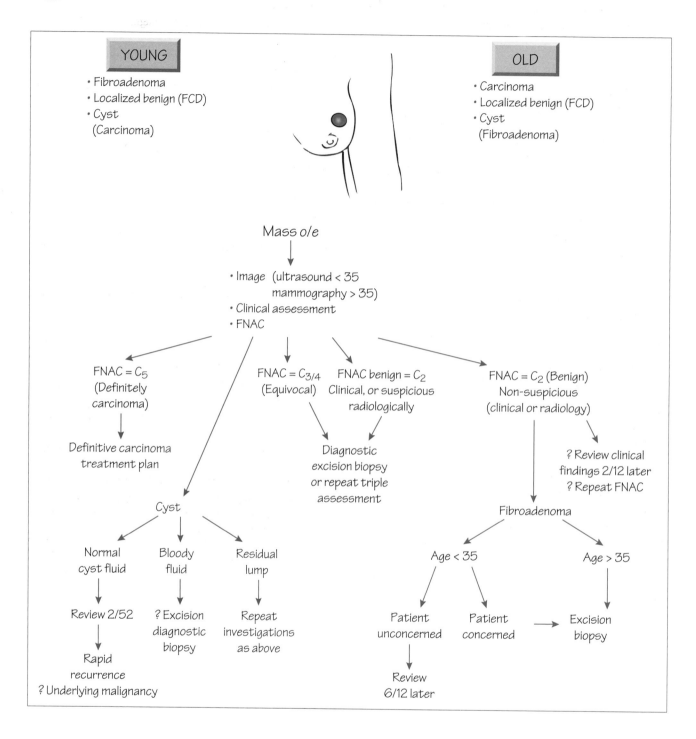

YOUNG

- Fibroadenoma
- Localized benign (FCD)
- Cyst
  (Carcinoma)

OLD

- Carcinoma
- Localized benign (FCD)
- Cyst
  (Fibroadenoma)

Mass o/e

- Image (ultrasound < 35
            mammography > 35)
- Clinical assessment
- FNAC

FNAC = C_5
(Definitely
carcinoma)

FNAC = $C_{3/4}$
(Equivocal)

FNAC benign = C_2
Clinical, or suspicious
radiologically

FNAC = C_2 (Benign)
Non-suspicious
(clinical or radiology)

Definitive carcinoma
treatment plan

Diagnostic
excision biopsy
or repeat triple
assessment

? Review clinical
findings 2/12 later
? Repeat FNAC

Cyst

Fibroadenoma

Normal
cyst fluid

Bloody
fluid

Residual
lump

Age < 35

Age > 35

Review 2/52

? Excision
diagnostic
biopsy

Repeat
investigations
as above

Patient
unconcerned

Patient
concerned

Excision
biopsy

Rapid
recurrence
? Underlying malignancy

Review
6/12 later

Definition

A breast lump is defined as any palpable mass in the breast. A breast lump is the most common presentation of both benign and malignant breast disease. Enlargement of the whole breast can occur either uni- or bilaterally, but this is not strictly a breast lump.

Key points

- The most common breast lumps occurring under the age of 35 years are fibroadenomas and fibrocystic disease.
- The most common breast lumps occurring over the age of 50 years are carcinomas and cysts.
- Pain is more characteristic of infection/inflammation than tumours.
- Skin/chest wall tethering is more characteristic of tumours than benign disease.
- Multiple lesions are usually benign (cysts or fibrocystic disease).

Differential diagnosis

Swelling of the whole breast

Bilateral

- Pregnancy, lactation.
- Idiopathic hypertrophy.
- Drug induced (e.g. stilboestrol, cimetidine).

Unilateral

- Enlargement in the newborn.
- Puberty.

Localized swellings in the breast

Mastitis/breast abscess

- During lactation: red, hot, tender lump, systemic upset.
- Tuberculous abscess: chronic, 'cold', recurrent, discharging sinus.

Cysts

- Galactocele: more common postpartum, tender but not inflamed, milky contents.
- Fibrocystic disease: irregular, ill defined, often tender.

Solid lumps

Benign include:

- Fibroadenoma: discrete, firm, well defined, regular, highly mobile.
- Fat necrosis: irregular, ill defined, hard, ?skin tethering.
- Lipoma: well defined, soft, non-tender, fairly mobile.
- Cystosarcoma phylloides: wide surgical excision (10% are malignant).

Malignant include:

- Carcinoma
  early: ill defined, hard, irregular, skin tethering
  late: spreading fixity, ulceration, fungation, '*peau d'orange*'.

Swellings behind the breast

- Rib deformities, chondroma, costochondritis (Tietze's disease).

Key investigations

- FNAC: tumours, fibroadenoma, fibrocystic disease, fat necrosis, mastitis.
- Ultrasound: fibroadenoma, cysts, tumours (best for young women/dense breasts).
- Mammography: tumours, cysts, fibrocystic disease, fat necrosis.
- Biopsy ('Trucut'/open surgical): usually provides definitive histology (may be radiologically guided if lump is small or impalpable—detected by mammography as part of breast screening programme).

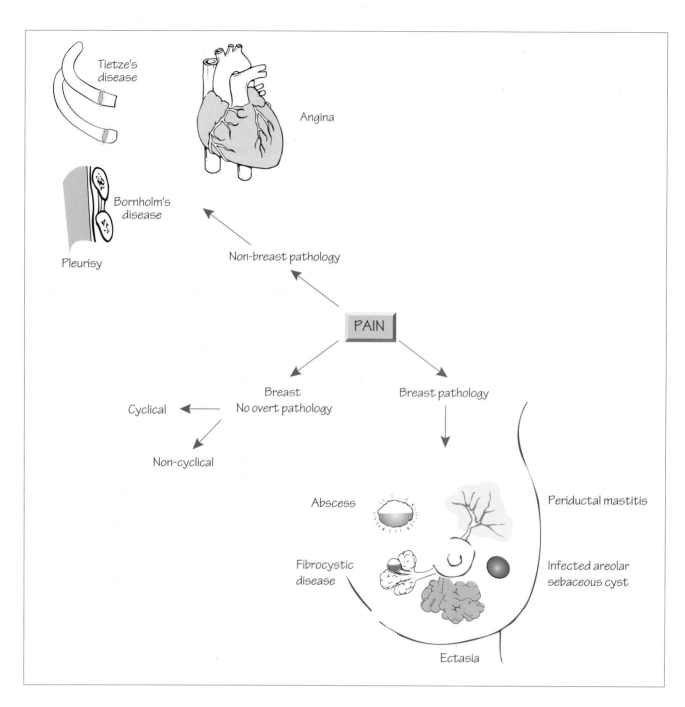

Definition

Mastalgia is any pain felt in the breast. *Cyclical mastalgia* is pain in the breast that varies in association with the menstrual cycle. *Non-cyclical mastalgia* is pain in the breast that follows no pattern or is intermittent.

Key points

- Mastalgia is commonly due to disorders of the breast or nipple tissue but may also be due to problems in the underlying chest wall or overlying skin.
- Pain is an uncommon presenting feature of tumours but any underlying mass should be investigated as for a mass (see Chapter 4).
- Always look for an associated infection in the breast.
- Mammography should be routine in women presenting over the age of 45 years to help exclude occult carcinoma.

Important diagnostic features

Non-breast conditions

- Tietze's disease (costochondritis): tenderness over medial ends of ribs, not limited to the breast area of the chest wall, relieved by NSAIDs.
- Bornholm's disease (epidemic pleurodynia): marked pain with no physical signs in the breast, worse with inspiration, no chest disease underlying, relieved with NSAIDs.
- Pleurisy: associated chest infection, pleural rub, may be bilateral.
- Angina: usually atypical angina, may be hard to diagnose, previous history of associated vascular disease.

Mastalgia due to breast pathology

Mastitis/breast abscess

- During lactation: red, hot, tender lump, systemic upset.
  Treatment: aspirate abscess (may need to be repeated), do not stop breast feeding, oral antibiotics.

- Non-lactational abscesses: recurrent, associated with smoking, associated with underlying ductal ectasia.
  Treatment: aspirate or incise and drain abscess, give oral antibiotics, stop smoking, prophylactic metronidazole for recurrent sepsis.

Infected sebaceous cyst

Single lump superficially in the skin of the periareolar region, previous history of painless cystic lump.
  Treatment: excise infected cyst.

Fibrocystic disease

Irregular, ill defined, may be associated lumps, tender more than very painful.

Mastalgia without breast pathology

- Pain often felt throughout the breast, often worse in the axillary tail, moderately tender to examination.
  Treatment for cyclical mastalgia: γ linoleic acid (evening primrose oil), danazol, tamoxifen.
  Treatment for non-cyclical mastalgia: NSAIDs, γ linoleic acid.

Key investigations

Non-breast origin

Chest X-ray, ECG (exercise)

Breast pathology

- FNAC (MC+S): associated palpable lump, ?fibrocystic disease, ?mastitis/abscess.
- Ultrasound (young women/dense breasts) or mammography (older women/small breasts).

Mastalgia without breast pathology

Mammography in women over 45 years

6 Nipple discharge

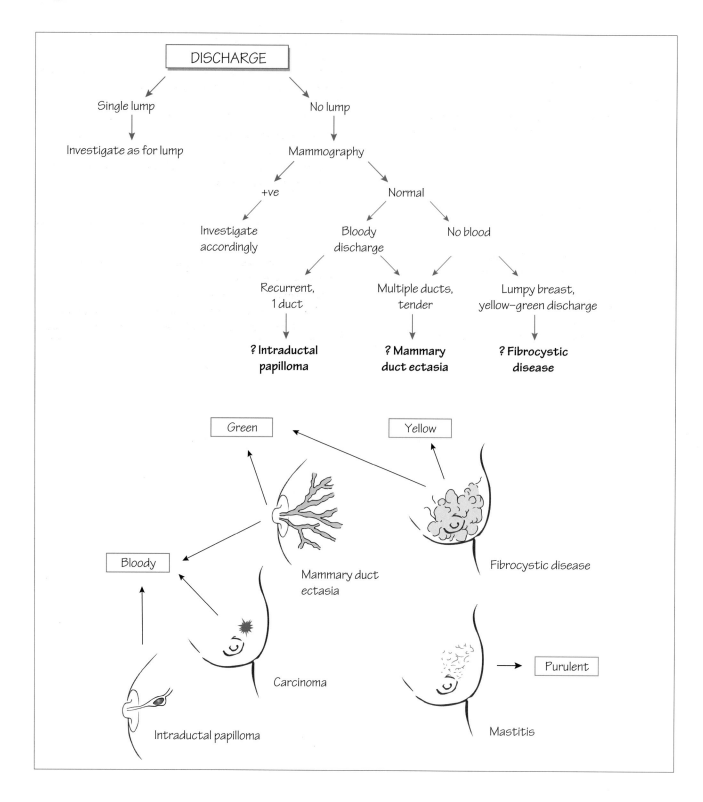

Definition

Any fluid (which may be physiological or pathological) emanating from the nipple.

Key points

- Milky discharge is rarely pathological.
- Purulent discharge is usually benign.
- Bloody discharge is often associated with neoplasia.
- If a lump is present, always investigate 'for the lump' rather than 'for the discharge'.

Differential diagnosis

Physiological discharges

Milky or clear

- Lactation.
- Lactorrhoea in the newborn ('witches' milk').
- Lactorrhoea at puberty (may be in either sex).

Pathological discharges

Serous yellow–green

- Fibrocystic disease: cyclical, tender, lumpy breasts.
- Mammary duct ectasia: usually multiple ducts, intermittent, may be associated with low-grade mastitis.

Bloody

- Duct papilloma: single duct, ?retro-areolar, 'pea-sized' lump.
- Carcinoma: ?palpable lump.
- Mammary duct ectasia: usually multiple ducts, intermittent, may be associated with low-grade mastitis.

Pus ± milk

- Acute suppurative mastitis: tender, swollen, hot breast, multiple ducts discharging.
- Tuberculous (rare): chronic discharge, periareolar fistulae, 'sterile' cultures on normal media.

Key investigations

- MC+S: acute mastitis, TB (Lowenstein–Jensen medium, Ziehl–Neelsen stains).
- Discharge cytology: carcinoma.
- Mammography: tumours, fibrocystic disease, ?ectasia.
- Ductal excision: may be needed for exclusion of neoplasia.

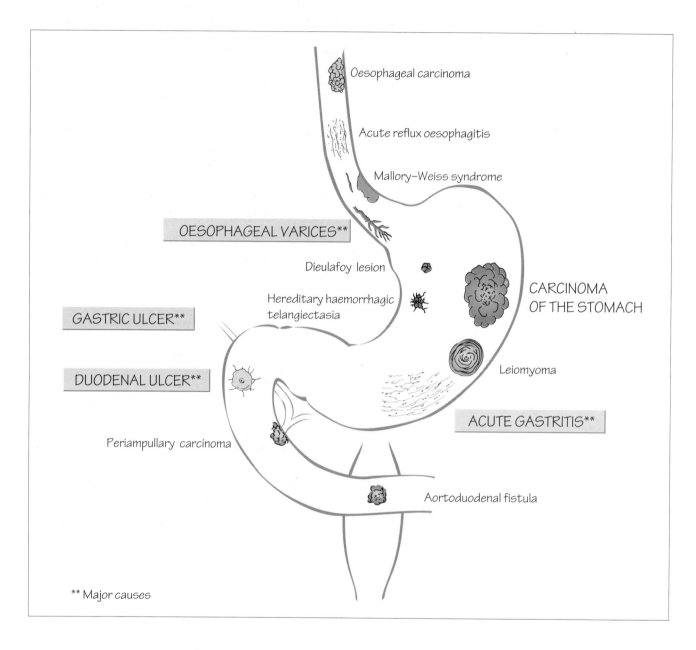

Oesophageal carcinoma

Acute reflux oesophagitis

Mallory–Weiss syndrome

OESOPHAGEAL VARICES**

Dieulafoy lesion

Hereditary haemorrhagic
telangiectasia

GASTRIC ULCER**

DUODENAL ULCER**

CARCINOMA
OF THE STOMACH

Leiomyoma

ACUTE GASTRITIS**

Periampullary carcinoma

Aortoduodenal fistula

** Major causes

Definitions

GI bleeding is any blood loss from the GI tract (from the mouth to the anus), which may present with haematemesis, melaena, rectal bleeding or anaemia. *Haematemesis* is defined as vomiting blood and is usually caused by upper GI disease. *Melaena* is the passage PR of a black treacle-like stool that contains altered blood, usually as a result of proximal bowel bleeding.

Key points

- Haematemesis is usually caused by lesions proximal to the duodeno-jejunal junction.
- Melaena may be caused by lesions anywhere from oesophagus to colon (upper GI lesions can cause frank PR bleeding).
- Most tumours more commonly cause anaemia than frank haematemesis.
- In young adults, PUD, congenital lesions and varices are common causes.
- In the elderly, tumours, PUD and angiodysplasia are common causes.

Important diagnostic features

Oesophagus

- Reflux oesophagitis: small volumes, bright red, associated with regurgitation.
- Oesophageal carcinoma (rare): scanty, blood-stained debris, rarely significant volume, associated with weight loss, anergia, dysphagia.
- Bleeding varices: sudden onset, painless, large volumes, dark red blood, history of (alcoholic) liver disease, physical findings of portal hypertension.
- Trauma during vomiting (Mallory–Weiss syndrome): bright red bloody vomit usually preceded by several normal but forceful vomiting episodes.

Stomach

- Erosive gastritis: small volumes, bright red, may follow alcohol or NSAID intake/stress, history of dyspeptic symptoms.
- Gastric ulcer: often larger-sized bleed, painless, possible herald smaller bleeds, accompanied by altered blood ('coffee grounds'), history of PUD.
- Gastric cancer: rarely large bleed, anaemia more common, associated weight loss, anorexia, dyspeptic symptoms.
- Gastric leiomyoma (rare): spontaneous-onset moderate-sized bleed.
- Dieulafoy's disease (rare): younger patients, spontaneous large bleed, difficult to diagnose.

Duodenum

- Duodenal ulcer: past history of duodenal ulcer, melaena often also prominent, symptoms of back pain, hunger pains, NSAID use.
- Aortoduodenal fistula (rare): usually infected graft post AAA repair, massive haematemesis and PR bleed, usually fatal.

Key investigations

- FBC: carcinomas, reflux oesophagitis.
- LFTs: liver disease (varices).
- Clotting: alcohol, bleeding diatheses.
- OGD: investigation of choice. High diagnostic accuracy, allows therapeutic manoeuvres also (varices: injection; ulcers: injection/cautery).
- Angiography: rare duodenal causes, obscure recurrent bleeds.
- Barium meal and follow through: useful for patients who are unfit for OGD (respiratory disease) and ?proximal jejunal lesions.

Essential management

8 Dyspepsia

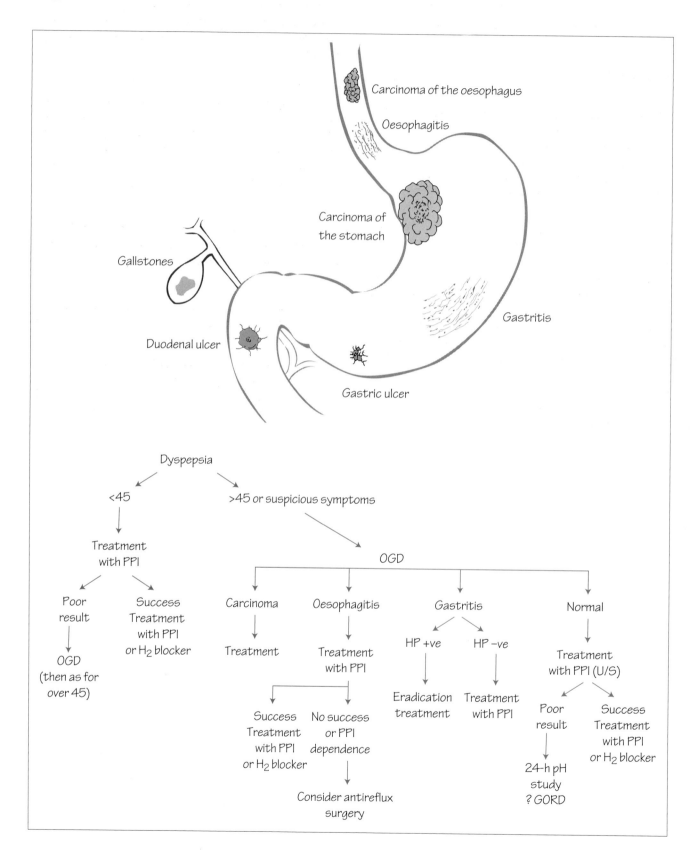

Definition

Dyspepsia is the feeling of discomfort or pain in the upper abdomen or lower chest. *Indigestion* may be used by the patient to mean dyspepsia, regurgitation symptoms or flatulence.

Key points

- Dyspepsia may be the only presenting symptom of upper GI malignancy. All older patients and patients with atypical history should have endoscopy.
- In young adults, gastro-oesophageal reflux and *Helicobacter*-positive gastritis are common causes.
- Dyspepsia is rarely the only symptom of gallstones—they are more often incidental findings.

Differential diagnosis

Oesophagus

- Reflux oesophagitis: retrosternal dyspepsia, worse after large meal/lying down, associated symptoms of regurgitation, pain on swallowing.
- Oesophageal carcinoma: new-onset dyspepsia in older patient, associated symptoms of weight loss/dysphagia/haematemesis, failure to respond to acid suppression treatment.

Stomach

- Gastritis: recurrent episodes of epigastric pain, transient or short-lived symptoms, may be associated with diet, responds well to antacids/acid suppression.

- Gastric ulcer: typically chronic epigastric pain, worse with food, 'food fear' may lead to weight loss, exacerbated by smoking/alcohol, occasionally relieved by vomiting.
- Carcinoma stomach: progressive symptoms, associated weight loss/anorexia, iron-deficient anaemia common, early satiety, epigastric mass.

Duodenum

- Duodenal ulcer: epigastric and back pain, chronic exacerbations lasting several weeks, relieved by food especially milky drinks, relieved by bed rest, more common in younger men, associated with *Helicobacter* infection.
- Duodenitis: often transient, mild symptoms only, associated with alcohol and smoking.

Gallstones

Dyspepsia is rarely the only symptom, associated RUQ pain, needs normal OGD and positive ultrasound to be considered as cause for dyspeptic symptoms.

Key investigations

- FBC: anaemia suggests malignancy.
- OGD: tumours, PUD, assessment of oesophagitis.
- 24-hour pH monitoring: ?GORD.
- Ultrasound: ?gallstones.

9 Vomiting

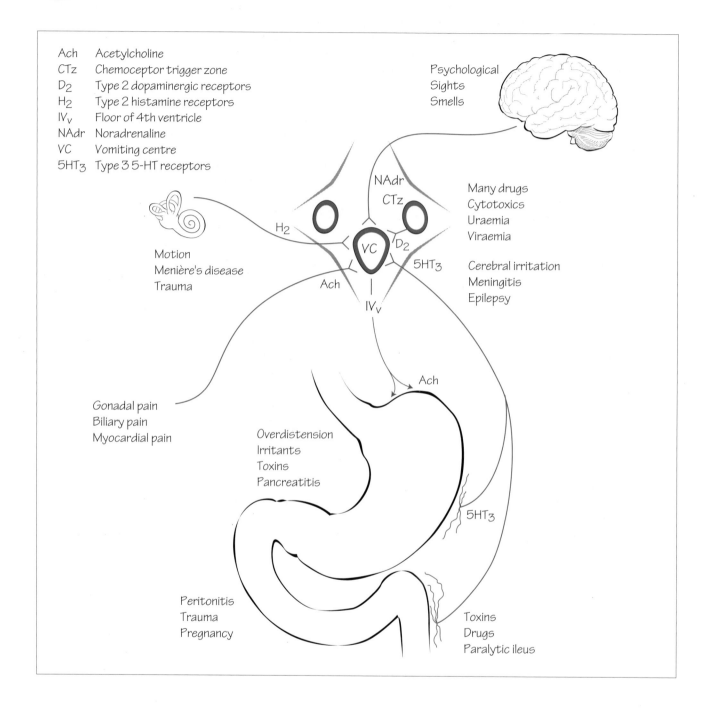

Ach	Acetylcholine
CTz	Chemoceptor trigger zone
D_2	Type 2 dopaminergic receptors
H_2	Type 2 histamine receptors
IV_v	Floor of 4th ventricle
NAdr	Noradrenaline
VC	Vomiting centre
$5HT_3$	Type 3 5-HT receptors

Psychological
Sights
Smells

NAdr
CTz

Many drugs
Cytotoxics
Uraemia
Viraemia

H_2

D_2

VC

$5HT_3$

Cerebral irritation
Meningitis
Epilepsy

Motion
Menière's disease
Trauma

Ach

IV_v

Ach

Gonadal pain
Biliary pain
Myocardial pain

Overdistension
Irritants
Toxins
Pancreatitis

$5HT_3$

Peritonitis
Trauma
Pregnancy

Toxins
Drugs
Paralytic ileus

Definitions

Vomiting is defined as the involuntary return to, and forceful expulsion from, the mouth of all or part of the contents of the stomach. *Waterbrash* is the sudden secretion and accumulation of saliva in the mouth as a reflex associated with dyspepsia. *Retching* is the process whereby forceful contractions of the diaphragm and abdominal muscles occur without evacuation of the stomach contents.

Key points

- Vomiting is initiated when the vomiting centre in the medulla oblongata is stimulated, either directly (central vomiting) or via various afferent fibres (reflex vomiting).
- Vomiting of different origins is mediated by different pathways and transmitters. Therapy is best directed according to cause.
- Consider mechanical causes (e.g. gastric outflow or intestinal obstruction) before starting therapy.

Important diagnostic features

Central vomiting

- Drugs, e.g. morphine sulphate, chemotherapeutic agents.
- Uraemia.
- Viral hepatitis.
- Hypercalcaemia of any cause.
- Acute infections, especially in children.
- Pregnancy.

Reflex vomiting

Gastrointestinal causes (5HT$_3$ and Ach mediated—treatment: promotilants, 5HT$_3$ antagonists)

- Ingestion of irritants.
  Bacteria, e.g. salmonella (gastroenteritis).
  Emetics, e.g. zinc sulphate, ipecacuanha.
  Drugs, e.g. alcohol, salicylates (gastritis).
  Poisons, e.g. salt, arsenic, phosphorus.
- PUD: especially gastric ulcer; vomiting relieves the pain.
- Intestinal obstruction.
  Hour-glass stomach (carcinoma of the stomach).
  Pyloric stenosis—infant: hypertrophic pyloric stenosis, projectile vomiting; adult: pyloric outlet obstruction secondary to PUD or malignant disease.
  Small bowel obstruction: adhesions, hernia, neoplasm, Crohn's disease.
  Large bowel obstruction: malignancy, volvulus, diverticular disease.
- Inflammation: appendicitis, peritonitis, pancreatitis, cholecystitis, biliary colic.

General causes (ACh and D$_2$ mediated—treatment: anticholinergics, antidopaminergics)

- Myocardial infarction.
- Ovarian disease, ectopic pregnancy.
- Severe pain (e.g. kick to the testis, gonadal torsion, blow to the epigastrium).
- Severe coughing (e.g. pulmonary TB, pertussis).

CNS causes (NAdr and ACh mediated—treatment: anticholinergics, sedatives)

- Raised intracranial pressure.
  Head injury.
  Cerebral tumour or abscess.
  Hydrocephalus.
  Meningitis.
  Cerebral haemorrhage.
- Migraine.
- Epilepsy.
- Offensive sights, tastes and smells.
- Hysteria.
- Middle ear disorders (H$_2$ mediated—treatment: antihistamines).
  Ménière's disease.
  Travel/motion sickness.

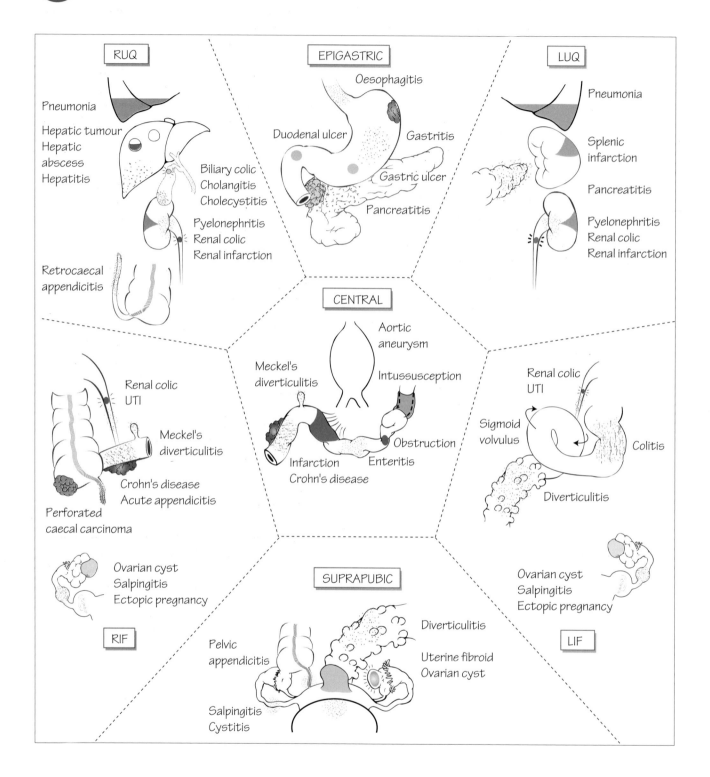

RUQ

Pneumonia

Hepatic tumour
Hepatic abscess
Hepatitis

Biliary colic
Cholangitis
Cholecystitis

Pyelonephritis
Renal colic
Renal infarction

Retrocaecal appendicitis

EPIGASTRIC

Oesophagitis

Duodenal ulcer

Gastritis

Gastric ulcer

Pancreatitis

LUQ

Pneumonia

Splenic infarction

Pancreatitis

Pyelonephritis
Renal colic
Renal infarction

CENTRAL

Aortic aneurysm

Meckel's diverticulitis

Intussusception

Obstruction

Infarction   Enteritis
Crohn's disease

Renal colic
UTI

Meckel's diverticulitis

Crohn's disease
Acute appendicitis

Perforated caecal carcinoma

Renal colic
UTI

Sigmoid volvulus

Colitis

Diverticulitis

Ovarian cyst
Salpingitis
Ectopic pregnancy

RIF

SUPRAPUBIC

Pelvic appendicitis

Diverticulitis

Uterine fibroid
Ovarian cyst

Salpingitis
Cystitis

Ovarian cyst
Salpingitis
Ectopic pregnancy

LIF

Definitions

Abdominal pain is a subjective unpleasant sensation felt in any of the abdominal regions. *Acute* abdominal pain is usually used to refer to pain of sudden onset, and/or short duration. *Referred pain* is the perception of pain in an area remote from the site of origin of the pain.

Key points

- The level of abdominal pain generally relates to the origin: foregut—upper; midgut—middle; hindgut—lower.
- Generally, colicky (visceral) pain is caused by stretching or contracting a hollow viscus (e.g. gallbladder, ureter, ileum).
- Generally, constant localized (somatic) pain is caused by peritoneal irritation and indicates the presence of inflammation/infection (e.g. pancreatitis, cholecystitis, appendicitis).
- Associated back pain suggests retroperitoneal pathology (aortic aneurysm, pancreatitis, posterior DU, pyelonephritis).
- Associated sacral or perineal pain suggests pelvic pathology (ovarian cyst, PID, pelvic abscess).
- Generally, very severe pain indicates ischaemia or generalized peritonitis (e.g. mesenteric infarction, perforated DU).
- Pain out of proportion to the physical signs suggests ischaemia without perforation.
- Remember referred causes of pain: pneumonia (right lower lobe), myocardial infarction, lumbar nerve root pathology.

Key investigations

FBC: leucocytosis, infective/inflammatory diseases, anaemia, occult malignancy, PUD.
- LFTs: usually abnormal in cholangitis, may be abnormal in acute cholecystitis.
- Amylase: serum level >3× upper limit of normal range is diagnostic of pancreatitis. Serum level 2–3× upper limit of normal range, ?pancreatitis, perforated ulcer, bowel ischaemia, severe sepsis. Serum level raised mildly (up to 2×) non-specific indicator of pathology.
- β-HCG (serum): ectopic pregnancy (serum level is more accurate than urinary hormone).
- Arterial blood gases: metabolic acidosis—?bowel ischaemia, peritonitis, pancreatitis.
- MSU: urinary tract infection (++ve nitrites, blood, protein), renal stone (++ve blood).
- ECG: myocardial infarction.
- Chest X-ray: perforated viscus (free gas), pneumonia.
- Abdominal X-ray:
  ischaemic bowel (dilated, thickened oedematous loops)
  pancreatitis ('sentinel' dilated upper jejunum)
  cholangitis (air in biliary tree)
  acute colitis (dilated, oedematous, featureless colon)
  acute obstruction (dilated loops, 'string of pearls' sign)
  renal stones (radiodense opacity in renal tract).
- Ultrasound:
  intra-abdominal abscesses (diverticular, appendicular, pelvic)
  acute cholecystitis/empyema
  ovarian pathology (cyst, ectopic pregnancy)
  trauma (liver/spleen haematoma)
  renal infections.
- OGD:
  PUD, gastritis.
- CT scan: is the investigation of choice for: undiagnosed peritoneal inflammation (particularly in the elderly where the differential diagnosis is wide, patients where laparotomy is considered and the diagnosis is uncertain), pancreatitis, trauma (liver/spleen/mesenteric injuries), diverticulitis, leaking aortic aneurysm.
- IVU: renal stones, renal tract obstruction.

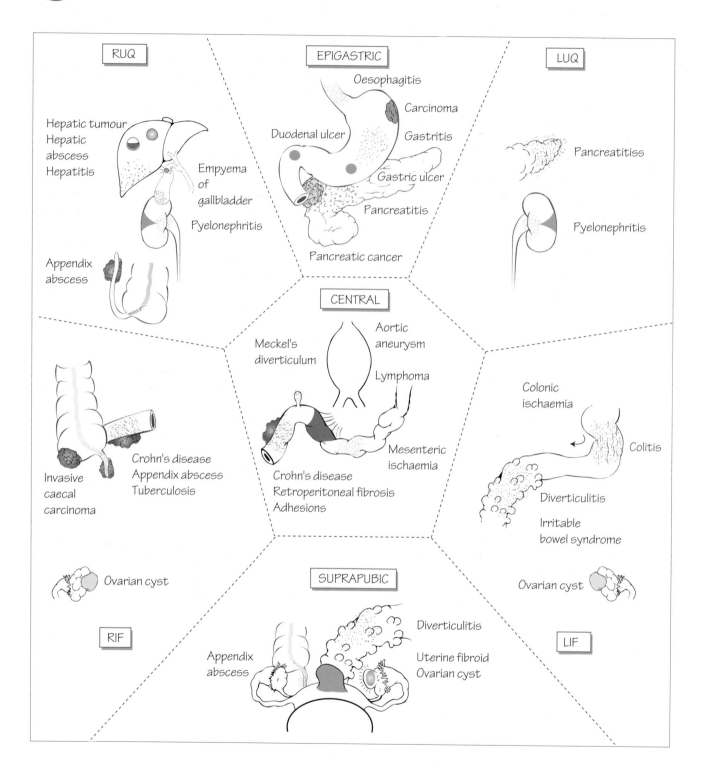

RUQ
EPIGASTRIC
LUQ

Hepatic tumour
Hepatic abscess
Hepatitis

Empyema of gallbladder

Pyelonephritis

Appendix abscess

Oesophagitis
Carcinoma
Duodenal ulcer
Gastritis
Gastric ulcer
Pancreatitis
Pancreatic cancer

Pancreatitiss
Pyelonephritis

CENTRAL

Meckel's diverticulum
Aortic aneurysm
Lymphoma
Mesenteric ischaemia

Invasive caecal carcinoma
Crohn's disease
Appendix abscess
Tuberculosis

Crohn's disease
Retroperitoneal fibrosis
Adhesions

Colonic ischaemia
Colitis
Diverticulitis
Irritable bowel syndrome

Ovarian cyst

SUPRAPUBIC

Ovarian cyst

RIF

Appendix abscess

Diverticulitis
Uterine fibroid
Ovarian cyst

LIF

Definition

Chronic abdominal pain is usually used to refer to pain that is either longstanding, of prolonged duration or of recurrent/intermittent nature. Chronic pain may be associated with acute exacerbations.

Key points

- Chronic abdominal pain of prolonged duration requires investigation.
- Adhesions as a cause of chronic abdominal pain should be a diagnosis of exclusion.
- Irritable bowel syndrome is less common than supposed—any atypical bowel symptoms should be investigated fully before diagnosing IBS.
- Back pain suggests a retroperitoneal origin.
- Sacral pain suggests a pelvic origin.
- Relationship to food strongly suggests a physical pathology and requires investigation.

Important diagnostic features

Irritable bowel syndrome

- Syndrome of colicky abdominal pain, bloating, hard pellety or watery stools, sensation of incomplete evacuation, often associated with frequency and urgency.
- Blood, mucus, abdominal physical findings, weight loss or recent onset of symptoms or onset in old age should suggest an organic cause and require thorough investigation.

Adhesions

- Associated with several syndromes of chronic or recurrent abdominal symptoms.
- **Adhesional abdominal pain**: difficult to diagnosis with any confidence, usually a diagnosis of exclusion, may be suggested by small bowel enema showing evidence of delayed transit or fixed strictures, rarely responds well to surgery.
- **Recurrent incomplete small bowel obstruction**: transient episodes of obstructive symptoms, often do not have all classical signs or symptoms present, abdominal signs may be unremarkable, self limiting.

Mesenteric angina

Classically occurs shortly after eating in elderly patients, colicky central abdominal pain, vomiting, food fear and weight loss. Usually associated with other occlusive vascular disease.

Meckel's diverticulum

May cause undiagnosed central abdominal pain in young adults. Occasionally associated with obscure PR bleeding, anaemia. Best diagnosed by radionuclide scanning.

Key investigations

- FBC: leucocytosis—chronic infective/inflammatory diseases, anaemia—occult malignancy, PUD, lymphocytosis—lymphoma.
- LFTs: common bile duct gallstones, hepatitis, liver tumours (primary/secondary).
- MSU: urinary tract infection (++ve nitrites, blood, protein), renal stone (++ve blood).
- ECG: ischaemic heart disease.
- Abdominal X-ray: chronic pancreatitis (small calcification throughout gland):
- Ultrasound:
  intra-abdominal abscesses (diverticular, appendicular, pelvic, hepatic)
  'gallstones', 'chronic cholecystitis'
  ovarian pathology (cyst)
  aortic aneurysm, renal tumours.
- OGD: PUD, gastritis, gastric or oesophageal carcinoma.
- Colonoscopy: diverticular disease, chronic colonic ischaemia.
- CT scan: chronic pancreatitis, pancreatic carcinoma, aortic aneurysm, retroperitoneal pathologies (fibrosis, lymphadenopathy, tumours).
- IVU: renal stones, renal tract tumours, renal tract obstruction.
- Visceral angiography/CT angiogram/Mesenteric MRA: mesenteric vascular disease.
- ERCP: chronic pancreatitis, pancreatic carcinoma.
- Small bowel enema: Crohn's disease, small bowel tumours, Meckel's diverticulum.
- Barium enema: ischaemic strictures, chronic colitis.

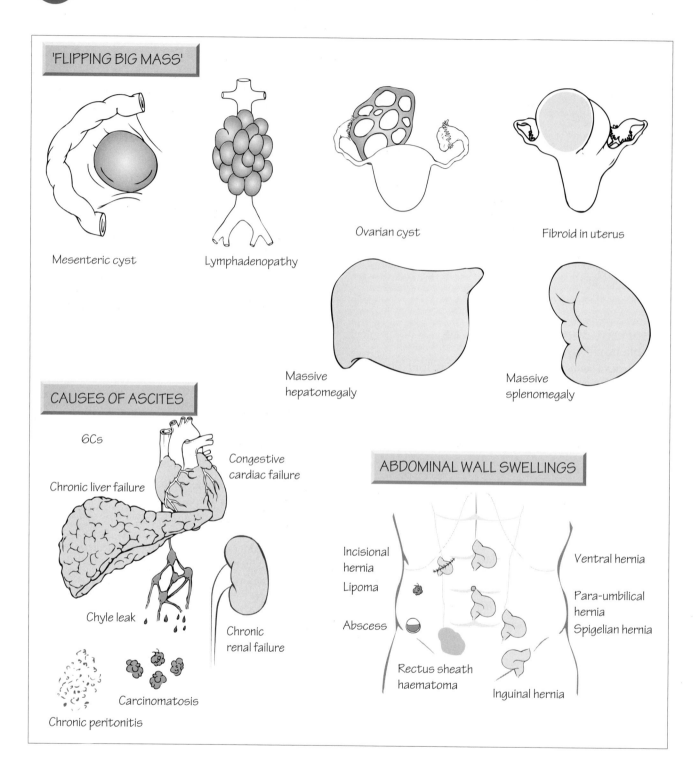

'FLIPPING BIG MASS'

Mesenteric cyst

Lymphadenopathy

Ovarian cyst

Fibroid in uterus

Massive hepatomegaly

Massive splenomegaly

CAUSES OF ASCITES

6Cs

Congestive cardiac failure

Chronic liver failure

Chyle leak

Chronic renal failure

Carcinomatosis

Chronic peritonitis

ABDOMINAL WALL SWELLINGS

Incisional hernia

Lipoma

Abscess

Rectus sheath haematoma

Inguinal hernia

Ventral hernia

Para-umbilical hernia

Spigelian hernia

Definition

An abdominal swelling is an abnormal protuberance that arises from the abdominal cavity or the abdominal wall and may be general or localized, acute or chronic, cystic or solid.

Key points

- Generalized abdominal swellings affect the entire abdominal cavity.
- Localized swellings can be located in the various regions of the abdomen.
- Abdominal wall swellings can be differentiated from intra-abdominal swellings by asking the patient to raise his or her head from the couch (intraperitoneal swellings disappear while abdominal wall swellings persist).
- Giant masses, other than ovarian cystadenocarcinoma, are rarely malignant.

Important diagnostic features

'Fat'

Obesity: deposition of fat in the abdominal wall and intra-abdominally (extraperitoneal layer, omentum and mesentery). Clinical obesity is present when a person's body weight is 120% greater than that recommended for their height, age and sex (body mass index).

'Flatus'

Intestinal obstruction: swallowed air accumulates in the bowel causing distension. This gives a tympanic note on percussion and produces the characteristic air–fluid levels and 'ladder' pattern on an abdominal radiograph. Sigmoid or caecal volvulus produces gross distension with characteristic features of distended loops on abdominal X-ray.

'Fluid'

- Intestinal obstruction: as well as air, fluid accumulates in the obstructed intestine.
- Ascites: fluid accumulates in the peritoneal cavity due to the '6 Cs':
- chronic peritonitis (e.g. tuberculosis, missed appendicitis)
- carcinomatosis (malignant deposits, especially ovary, stomach)
- chronic liver disease (cirrhosis, secondary deposits, portal or hepatic vein obstruction, parasitic infections)
- congestive heart failure (RVF)
- chronic renal failure (nephrotic syndrome)
- chyle (lymphatic duct disruption).

'Faeces'

Chronic constipation: faeces accumulate in the colon producing abdominal distension. Congenital causes include spina bifida and Hirschsprung's disease. Acquired causes include emotional disorders, chronic dehydration, drugs (opiates, anticholinergics, phenothiazines) and hypothyroidism.

'Fetus'

Pregnancy: swelling arises out of the pelvis.

'Flipping big mass'

Usually cystic lesions: giant ovarian cystadenoma, mesenteric cyst, retroperitoneal lymphadenopathy (lymphoma), giant uterine fibroid, giant splenomegaly, giant hepatomegaly, giant renal tumour, desmoid tumour.

Key investigations—*abdominal masses*

- FBC: lymphomas, infections.
- LFTs: liver disease.
- U+Es: renal disease.
- Abdominal X-ray:
  ascites ('ground glass' appearance, loss of visceral outlines)
  large mass (bowel gas pattern eccentric, paucity of gas in one quadrant)
  fibroid ('popcorn' calcification).
- Ultrasound: ascites, may show cystic masses.
- CT scan: investigation of choice, differentiates origin and relationships.
- Paracentesis: MC+S (infections), cytology (tumours).
- Liver biopsy: undiagnosed hepatomegaly.

Key investigation—*abdominal wall swellings*

- Ultrasound: subcutaneous lumps
- CT scan: abscesses, hernias
- Herniography: rarely used for possible hernias with negative other investigations
- Laparoscopy: diagnosis and possible treatment of hernia

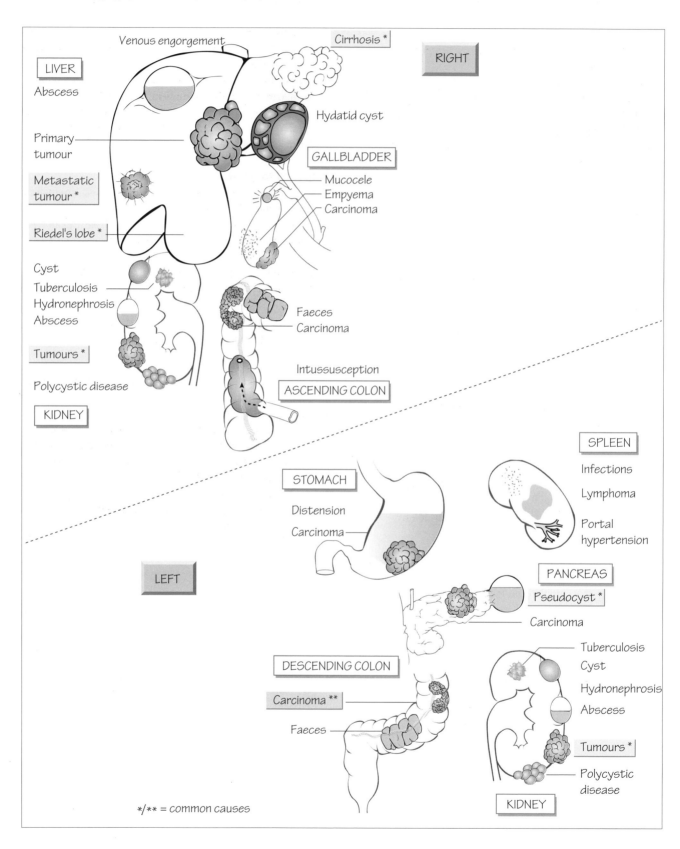

Venous engorgement

Cirrhosis *

RIGHT

LIVER

Abscess

Hydatid cyst

Primary tumour

GALLBLADDER

Mucocele
Empyema
Carcinoma

Metastatic tumour *

Riedel's lobe *

Cyst
Tuberculosis
Hydronephrosis
Abscess

Faeces
Carcinoma

Tumours *

Intussusception

ASCENDING COLON

Polycystic disease

KIDNEY

SPLEEN

Infections

Lymphoma

Portal hypertension

STOMACH

Distension

Carcinoma

LEFT

PANCREAS

Pseudocyst *

Carcinoma

Tuberculosis
Cyst
Hydronephrosis
Abscess

DESCENDING COLON

Carcinoma **

Tumours *

Faeces

Polycystic disease

KIDNEY

*/** = common causes

Key points

- Hepatic mass: moves with respiration, dull to percussion, cannot 'get above' it, enlarges/descends towards RIF.
- Splenic mass: moves with respiration, dull to percussion, cannot 'get above' it, enlarges/descends towards RIF, may have a notched border.
- Renal mass: moves somewhat with respiration, usually resonant due to overlying bowel gas, bimanually palpable (ballotable).
- Retroperitoneal mass: no movement with respiration, difficult to delineate, resonant to percussion.
- Bowel masses: often mobile, may be well defined.

Liver

- Riedel's lobe: smooth, non-tender, lateral/right lobe:, 'tongue-like', men < women.
- Infective hepatitis: smooth, tender, global enlargement.
- Liver abscess: usually one large abscess, ?amoebic, very tender, systemically unwell.
- Hydatid cyst: smooth, may be loculated, ?history of tropical travel.
- Venous congestion: smooth, tender, pulsatile (slightly irregular (cirrhotic) if chronic).
- Cirrhosis: irregular, firm, 'knobbly'.
- Tumours:
  primary: solitary, large, non-tender, ?lobulated
  secondary: often multiple, irregular, rock hard, centrally umbilicated.

Gallbladder

- Generally: oval, smooth, projects towards RIF, beneath the tip of the ninth rib, moves with respiration.
- Mucocele: large gallbladder, moderately tender, smooth walled.

- Empyema: acutely tender, difficult to palpate clearly because of pain.
- Carcinoma of gallbladder: nodular, hard, irregular.

Renal masses

- Perinephric abscess/pyonephrosis: acutely tender, systemic signs, rarely large.
- Hydronephrosis: large, smooth, tense kidney. May be massive.
- Solitary cyst: smooth, non-tender, may be massive.
- Polycystic disease: frequently very large, lobulated, smooth.
- Renal carcinoma: irregular, nodular, often hard, ?fixed.
- Nephroblastoma: large mass in children.

Suprarenal gland

- Generally: only palpable when large, moves with respiration, difficult to define borders.
- Adenomas: usually cystic if palpable.
- Infections: ?chronic fungal infections, may be tender, systemic features.
- Congenital hyperplasia: young children, endocrine disorders associated, smooth, non-tender.

Key investigations

- FBC: anaemia, tumours.
- WCC: lymphomas, Crohn's disease, appendicitis/diverticulitis.
- LFTs: liver lesions.
- Ultrasound: pancreatic (pseudo)cysts, aortic aneurysm.
- CT scan: pancreatic tumours, lymphadenopathy, retroperitoneal/mesenteric cysts, aortic aneurysm, omental deposits.
- Gastroscopy: stomach tumours.
- Colonoscopy: colonic tumours.
- Small bowel enema: small intestinal tumours.
- Barium enema: colonic tumours.

Abdominal swellings (localized): upper abdominal/2

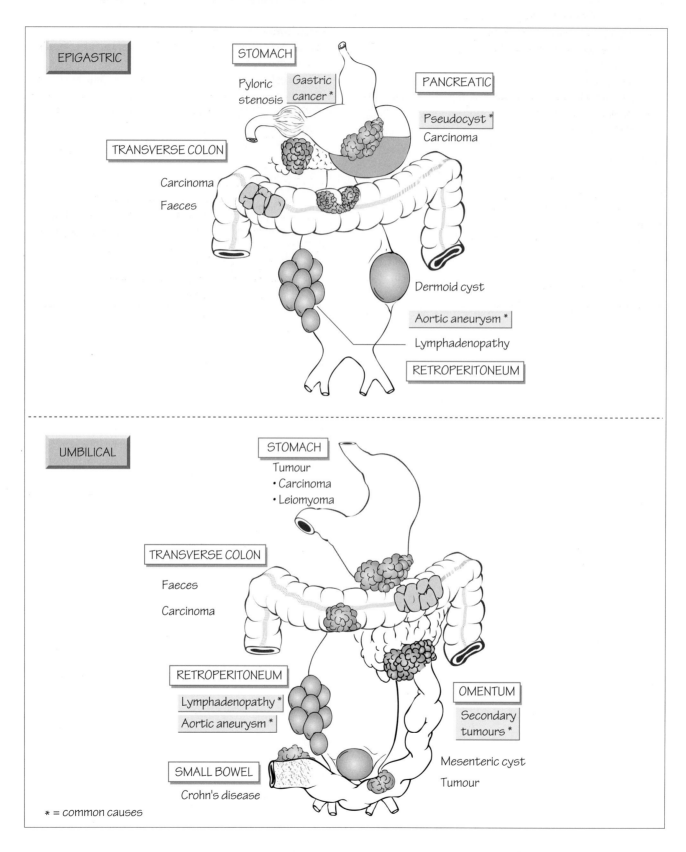

EPIGASTRIC

STOMACH

Pyloric stenosis   Gastric cancer *

PANCREATIC

Pseudocyst *
Carcinoma

TRANSVERSE COLON

Carcinoma

Faeces

Dermoid cyst

Aortic aneurysm *

Lymphadenopathy

RETROPERITONEUM

UMBILICAL

STOMACH
Tumour
• Carcinoma
• Leiomyoma

TRANSVERSE COLON

Faeces

Carcinoma

RETROPERITONEUM

Lymphadenopathy *

Aortic aneurysm *

OMENTUM

Secondary tumours *

Mesenteric cyst

Tumour

SMALL BOWEL

Crohn's disease

* = common causes

Colon

- Faeces: soft, putty-like mass, mobile, non-tender, can be indented.
- Carcinoma: firm-hard, irregular, non-tender, may be mobile (fixity strongly suggests carcinoma).
- Intussusception: mobile, smooth, sausage-shaped mass.

Stomach

- Gastric distension: soft, fluctuant, succussion splash present.
- Neoplasm: irregular, hard, craggy, immobile, does not descend on inspiration.

Pancreas

- Generally: does not move with respiration, fixed to retroperitoneum, poorly defined.
- Pseudocyst/cyst: mildly tender (worse if infected), symptoms of gastric obstruction.
- Carcinoma: hard, irregular, non-tender, fixed.

Retroperitoneum

- Lymphadenopathy: solid, immobile, irregular, 'rubbery', may be massive, particularly if lymphomatous.

- Dermoid cysts (rare): deep seated, smooth, recurrent after surgery.
- Aortic aneurysm: smooth, fusiform, pulsatile, expansile, may be tender.

Omentum

Secondary carcinoma: hard, irregular, mobile, 'pancake like', often ovarian carcinoma.

Key investigations

- FBC: anaemia, tumours.
- WCC: lymphomas, Crohn's disease, appendicitis/diverticulitis.
- LFTs: liver lesions.
- Ultrasound: pancreatic (pseudo)cysts, aortic aneurysm.
- CT scan: pancreatic tumours, lymphadenopathy, retroperitoneal/mesenteric cysts, aortic aneurysm, omental deposits.
- Gastroscopy: stomach tumours.
- Colonoscopy: colonic tumours.
- Small bowel enema: small intestinal tumours.
- Barium enema: colonic tumours.

---

14 Abdominal swellings (localized): lower abdominal

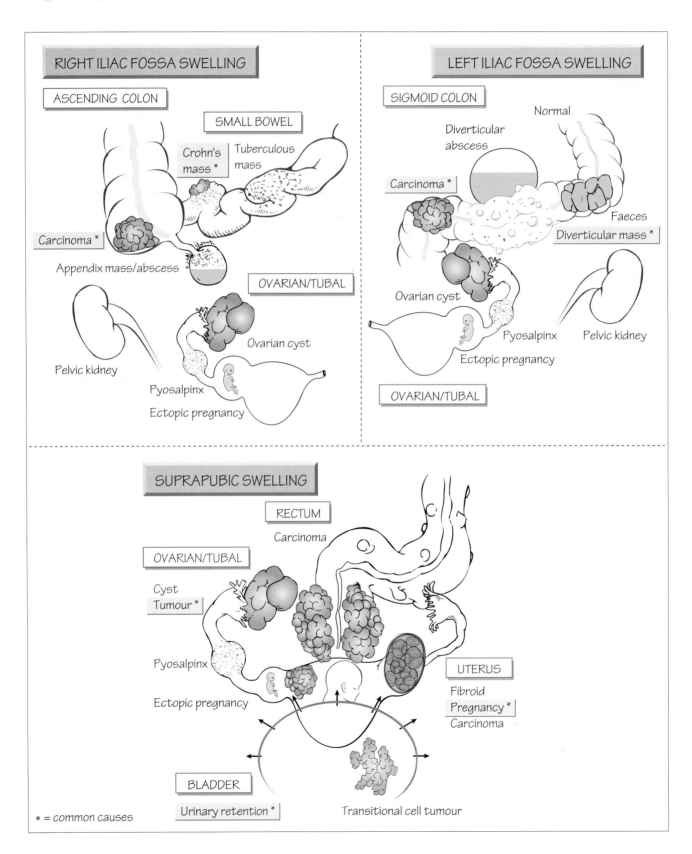

RIGHT ILIAC FOSSA SWELLING

ASCENDING COLON

SMALL BOWEL

Crohn's mass *   Tuberculous mass

Carcinoma *

Appendix mass/abscess

OVARIAN/TUBAL

Pelvic kidney

Ovarian cyst

Pyosalpinx

Ectopic pregnancy

LEFT ILIAC FOSSA SWELLING

SIGMOID COLON

Normal

Diverticular abscess

Carcinoma *

Faeces

Diverticular mass *

Ovarian cyst

Pyosalpinx   Pelvic kidney

Ectopic pregnancy

OVARIAN/TUBAL

SUPRAPUBIC SWELLING

RECTUM

Carcinoma

OVARIAN/TUBAL

Cyst
Tumour *

Pyosalpinx

Ectopic pregnancy

UTERUS

Fibroid
Pregnancy *
Carcinoma

BLADDER

Urinary retention *   Transitional cell tumour

* = common causes

Sigmoid colon

- Diverticular mass: tender, ill defined, rubbery hard, non-mobile.
- Paracolic abscess: acutely tender, ill defined, ?fluctuant, systemic upset.
- Carcinoma: hard, craggy, non-tender unless perforated, immobile, associated with altered bowel habit/obstructive symptoms.
- Faeces: firm, indentable/'malleable', mobile with colon.
- Normal: only in a thin person, non-tender, chord like.

Caecum/ascending colon

- Appendix mass/abscess: acutely tender, ill defined, ?fluctuant, systemic upset.
- Carcinoma: hard, craggy, non-tender unless perforated, immobile, associated with anaemia/weight loss and anergia.

Terminal ileum

- Crohn's mass: tender, ill defined, rubbery hard, non-mobile.
- Tuberculous mass: mildly tender, ill defined, firm, associated with cutaneous sinuses, ?systemic TB.

Ovary/fallopian tube

- Cyst: may be massive, usually mobile, ?bimanually palpable on PV examination.
- Neoplasm.
- Ectopic pregnancy: very tender, associated with PV bleeding/intra-abdominal bleeding and collapse.
- Salpingo-oophoritis: very tender, bimanually palpable, associated with PV discharge.

Bladder

- Generally: midline swelling, extends up towards umbilicus, dull to percussion, non-mobile, cannot 'get below' it.
- Retention of urine: stony dull to percussion, associated with desire to pass urine, disappears on voiding/catheterization.

- Transitional cell carcinoma: hard, irregular, fixed, may be associated with dysuria, haematuria and desire to pass urine on examination.

Uterus

- Pregnancy: smooth, regular, fetal heart sounds heard/movements!
- Fibromyoma: usually smooth, may be pedunculated and mobile, non-tender, associated menorrhagia.
- Uterine carcinoma: firm uterus, may be tender, irregular only if tumour is extrauterine, associated PV bloody discharge.

Rectum

Carcinoma: firm, irregular, non-tender, relatively immobile, associated alteration in bowel habit/PR bleeding.

Urachus (rare)

Cyst: small swelling in midline, ?associated umbilical discharge.

Other

Pelvic kidney: smooth, regular, non-tender, non-mobile.

Anatomy and normal bilirubin metabolism

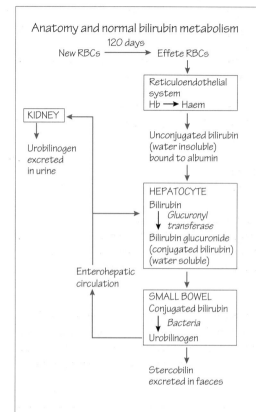

New RBCs → (120 days) → Effete RBCs

Reticuloendothelial system
Hb → Haem

KIDNEY
Urobilinogen excreted in urine

Unconjugated bilirubin (water insoluble) bound to albumin

HEPATOCYTE
Bilirubin
↓ *Glucuronyl transferase*
Bilirubin glucuronide (conjugated bilirubin) (water soluble)

Enterohepatic circulation

SMALL BOWEL
Conjugated bilirubin
↓ *Bacteria*
Urobilinogen

Stercobilin excreted in faeces

Biochemical features of different types of jaundice

Type of jaundice	Haemolytic	Hepatocellular Early	Late	Obstructive
Serum bilirubin				
Unconjugated	↑	N / ↑	N / ↑	N
Conjugated	N	N	↑	↑↑
Urinary bilirubin	N / ↑	↑	↑	↑↑
Urobilinogen	N / ↑	N	↓	↓↓
LFTs				
Alkaline phosphatase	N	N	↑	↑↑
γ-GT transaminase	N	↑	↑	↑↑
Transaminases	N	↑	↑↑	N / ↑
Lactate dehydrogenase	N	↑	↑↑	N / ↑
FBC				
Reticulocytes	> 2%	N	N	N

CAUSES OF OBSTRUCTIVE JAUNDICE

MURAL / INTRINSIC

Liver cell transport abnormalities
Sclerosing cholangitis
Cholangiocarcinoma
Mirrizi's syndrome (gallbladder mass associated with cholecystitis)
Benign stricture
• Postinflammatory
• Postoperative
• Postradiotherapy

INTRALUMINAL

Infestation
• Clonorchis
• Schistosomiasis
Gallstones

EXTRINSIC

Portal lymphadenopathy
Chronic pancreatitis
Pancreatic tumour
Ampullary tumour
Duodenal tumour

Definition

Jaundice (also called *icterus*) is defined as yellowing of the skin and sclera from accumulation of the pigment bilirubin in the blood and tissues. The bilirubin level has to exceed 35–40 mmol/l before jaundice is clinically apparent.

Key points

- Jaundice can be classified simply as pre-hepatic (haemolytic), hepatic (hepatocellular) and post-hepatic (obstructive).
- Most of the surgically treatable causes of jaundice are post-hepatic (obstructive).
- Painless progressive jaundice is highly likely to be due to malignancy.

Differential diagnosis

The following list explains the mechanisms behind the causes of jaundice.

Pre-hepatic/haemolytic jaundice

Haemolytic/congenital hyperbilirubinaemias

Excess production of unconjugated bilirubin exhausts the capacity of the liver to conjugate the extra load, e.g. haemolytic anaemias (e.g. hereditary spherocytosis, sickle cell disease, hypersplenism, thalassaemia).

Hepatic/hepatocellular jaundice

Hepatic unconjugated hyperbilirubinaemia

- Failure of transport of unconjugated bilirubin into the cell, e.g. Gilbert's syndrome.
- Failure of glucuronyl transferase activity, e.g. Crigler–Najjar syndrome.

Hepatic conjugated hyperbilirubinaemia

Hepatocellular injury. Hepatocyte injury results in failure of excretion of bilirubin, e.g.

> infections: viral hepatitis;
> poisons: CCl_4, aflatoxin;
> drugs: paracetamol, halothane.

Post-hepatic/obstructive jaundice

Post-hepatic conjugated hyperbilirubinaemia

Anything that blocks the release of conjugated bilirubin from the hepatocyte or prevents its delivery to the duodenum.

Courvoisier's law

'A palpable gallbladder in the presence of jaundice is unlikely to be due to gallstones.' It usually indicates the presence of a neoplastic stricture (tumour of pancreas, ampulla, duodenum, CBD), chronic pancreatitic stricture or portal lymphadenopathy.

Key investigations

- FBC: haemolysis.
- LFTs: alkaline phosphatase (cholestasis), γ-GT and transaminases (hepatocellular).
- Clotting: PT (elevated in cholestatic and hepatocellular jaundice).
- Urinary urobilinogen

Haemolytic
- Blood film
- Reticulocyte count
- Autoantibody screen

Hepatocellular
- Viral titres: including hepatitis A/B/C, CMV, EBV
- Ultrasound: details of hepatic parenchyma.
- Liver biopsy: hepatocellular disease

Obstructive
U/S CBD and gallbladder

CBD dilated / No gallstones
↓
?Ca pancreas/CBD
↓
ERCP +/– stent
CT scan/MRCP

CBD dilated / Gallstones
↓
ERCP
Surgery

Other cause found
↓
ERCP
CT scan
↓
Surgery

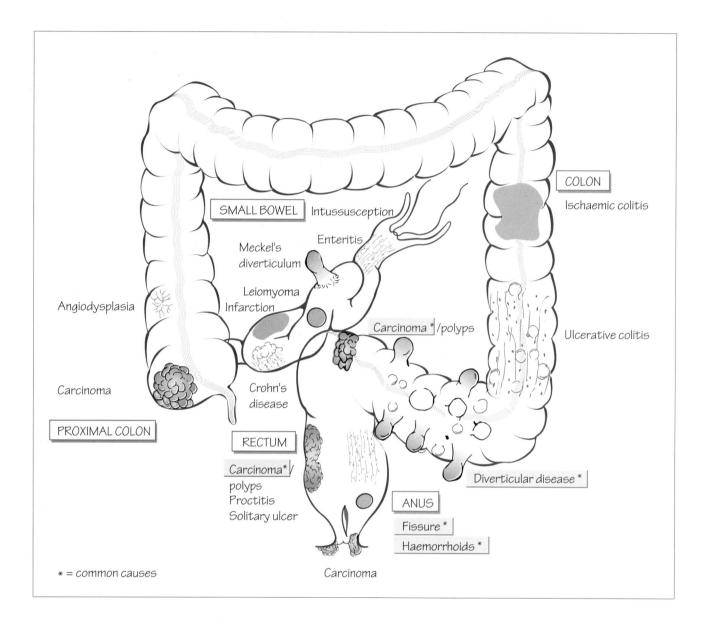

COLON
Ischaemic colitis

SMALL BOWEL Intussusception

Enteritis

Meckel's
diverticulum

Leiomyoma
Infarction

Angiodysplasia

Carcinoma */polyps

Ulcerative colitis

Carcinoma

Crohn's
disease

PROXIMAL COLON

RECTUM

Carcinoma*/
polyps
Proctitis
Solitary ulcer

Diverticular disease *

ANUS

Fissure *

Haemorrhoids *

* = common causes

Carcinoma

Key points

- Anorectal bleeding is characteristically bright red, associated with defaecation, not mixed with the stool and visible on toilet paper—often associated with other symptoms of anorectal disease.
- Distal (left-sided/sigmoid) bleeding is characteristically dark red, with clots, may be mixed with the stool.
- Proximal colonic or ileal bleeding is characteristically dark red, fully mixed with the stool or occult—unless heavy when it may appear as 'distal' or 'anorectal' in type.
- In children, acute anal fissure, Meckel's diverticulum, intussusception and ileal tumours are common causes.
- In young adults, colitis, Meckel's diverticulum, anal fissure and haemorrhoids are common causes.
- In the elderly, neoplasia, diverticular disease and angiodysplasia are common causes.
- Always do a rectal examination and rigid sigmoidoscopy in all patients.
- New rectal bleeding age >55 always deserves colonic investigation—never assume it is a simple anal cause.
- Bright red bleeding with no obvious anal cause requires at least a flexible sigmoidoscopy.
- Any suggestion of dark red blood or a +ve FOB requires colonic imaging or colonoscopy.

Important diagnostic features

Small intestine

- Meckel's diverticulum: young adults, painless bleeding, darker red/melaena common.
- Intussusception: young children, colicky abdominal pain, retching, bright red/mucus stool.
- Enteritis (infective/radiation/Crohn's).
- Ischaemic: severe abdominal pain, physical examination shows mesenteric ischaemia or AF, few signs, later collapse and shock.
- Tumours (leiomyoma/lymphoma): rare, intermittent history, often modest volumes lost.

Proximal colon

- Angiodysplasia: common in the elderly, painless, no warning, often large volume, fresh and clots mixed.
- Carcinoma of the caecum: more often causes anaemia than PR bleeding.

Colon

- Polyps/carcinoma: may be large volume or small, ?associated change in bowel habit, blood often mixed with stool.
- Diverticular disease: spontaneous onset, painless, large volume, mostly fresh blood, previous history of constipation.
- Ulcerative colitis: blood mixed with mucus, associated with systemic upset, long history, intermittent course, diarrhoea prominent.
- Ischaemic colitis: elderly, severe abdominal pain, AF, bloody diarrhoea, collapse and shock later.

Rectum

- Carcinoma of the rectum: change in bowel habit common, rarely large volumes.
- Proctitis: bloody mucus, purulent diarrhoea in infected, perianal irritation common.
- Solitary rectal ulcer: bleeding post-defaecation, small volumes, feeling of 'lump in anus', mucus discharge.

Anus

- Haemorrhoids: bright red bleeding post-defaecation, stops spontaneously, perianal irritation.
- Fissure -in-ano: extreme pain post-defaecation, small volumes bright red blood on stool and toilet paper.
- Carcinoma of the anus: elderly, mass in anus, small volumes bloody discharge, anal pain, unhealing ulcers.
- Perianal Crohn's disease.

Key investigations

- FBC: anaemia—tumours/chronic colitis.
- Clotting: bleeding diatheses.
- FOB: testing.
- PR/sigmoidoscopy: anorectal tumours, prolapse, haemorrhoids, distal colitis.
- Abdominal X-ray: intussusception.
- Flexible sigmoidoscopy: suspected colitis
- Colonoscopy: diverticular disease, colon tumours, angiodysplasia.
- Angiography: angiodysplasia, small bowel causes (especially Meckel's). (Needs active bleeding 0.5 ml/min, highly accurate when positive, invasive, allows embolization therapy.)
- Labelled RBC scan: angiodysplasia, small bowel causes, obscure colonic causes. (Needs active bleeding 1 ml/min, less accurate placement of source, non-invasive, non-therapeutic.)
- Small bowel enema: small bowel tumours.

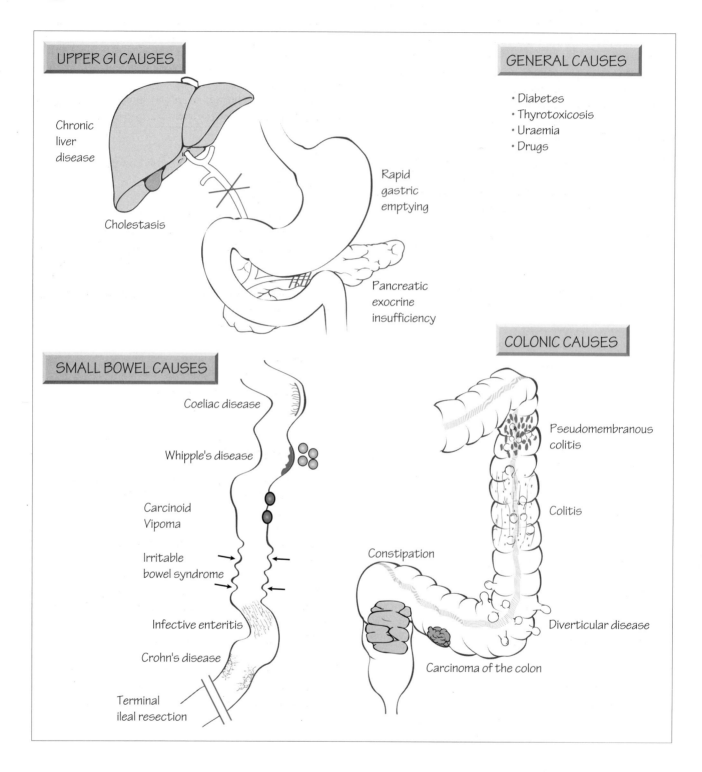

UPPER GI CAUSES

Chronic liver disease

Cholestasis

Rapid gastric emptying

Pancreatic exocrine insufficiency

GENERAL CAUSES

- Diabetes
- Thyrotoxicosis
- Uraemia
- Drugs

SMALL BOWEL CAUSES

Coeliac disease

Whipple's disease

Carcinoid
Vipoma

Irritable bowel syndrome

Infective enteritis

Crohn's disease

Terminal ileal resection

COLONIC CAUSES

Pseudomembranous colitis

Colitis

Constipation

Diverticular disease

Carcinoma of the colon

Definitions

Diarrhoea is defined as the passage of loose, liquid stool. *Urgency* is the sensation of the need to defaecate without being able to delay. It may indicate rectal irritability but also occurs where the volume of liquid stool is too large, causing the rectum to be overwhelmed as a storage vessel. *Frequency* merely reflects the number of stools passed and may or may not be associated with urgency or diarrhoea.

Key points

- Bloody diarrhoea is always pathological and usually indicates colitis of one form or another.
- Infective causes are common in acute transient diarrhoea.
- In diarrhoea of uncertain origin, remember the endocrine causes.
- Consider parasitic infections in a history of foreign travel.
- Alternating morning diarrhoea and normal/pellety stools later in the day is rarely pathological.
- Diarrhoea developing in hospitalized patients may be due to *Clostridium difficile* infection—check for CD toxin in the stool.

Important diagnostic features

Acute diarrhoea

Infections

- *Shigella/Salmonella*: associated colicky abdominal pain, vomiting.
- Dysentery: blood and mucus in motions, ulcers in rectum and *Entamoeba histolytica* in the stool, fever, sweating, tachycardia.
- Cholera: severe diarrhoea, 'rice water' stool, dehydration, history of foreign travel.
- *Giardiasis*.

Antibiotics

Short-lived, self-limiting, mild colicky pain.

Pseudomembranous colitis

Caused by *Clostridium difficile* infection, characterized by severe diarrhoea which may be bloody but occasionally acute constipation may indicate severe disease. Characteristic features on colonoscopy.

Chronic diarrhoea

Small bowel disease

- Crohn's disease: diarrhoea, pain prominent, blood and mucus less common, young adults, long history, chronic malnourishment and weight loss.
- Coeliac disease: history of wheat and cereals intolerance, may present in adulthood with chronic diarrhoea and weight loss, abdominal pains.
- 'Blind loop' syndrome: frothy, foul-smelling liquid stool, due to bacterial overgrowth and fermentation, usually associated with previous surgery, may complicate Crohn's disease.

Large bowel disease

- Ulcerative colitis: intermittent, blood and mucus, colicky pains, young adults. May be a short history in first presentations. Rarely presents with acute fulminant colitis with acute abdominal signs.
- Colon cancer: older, occasional blood streaks and mucus, change in frequency may be the only feature, positive faecal occult blood, rectal mass.
- Irritable bowel syndrome: diarrhoea and constipation mixed, bloating, colicky pain, small stool pellets, never blood.
- Spurious: impacted faeces in rectum, liquefied stool passes around faecal obstruction, elderly, mental illness, constipating drugs.
- Polyps (villous) (rare): watery, mucoid diarrhoea, K^+ loss, most common in rectum.
- Diverticular disease (rare).

Systemic disease

Thyrotoxicosis, anxiety, peptides from tumours (VIP, serotonin, substance P, calcitonin), laxative abuse.

Key investigations

- FBC: leucocytosis (infective causes, colitis), anaemia (colon cancer, ulcerative colitis, diverticular disease).
- Anti α-gliadin Abs: coeliac disease.
- Thyroid function tests: hyperthyroidism.
- Stool culture: infections (remember microscopy for parasites).
- Proctoscopy/sigmoidoscopy: cancer, colitis, polyps (simple, easy, cheap and safe; performed in outpatients).
- Flexible sigmoidoscopy: cancer, polyps, colitis, infections (relatively safe, well tolerated, high sensitivity).
- Colonoscopy: colitis (extent and severity), pseudomembranous colitis.
- Small bowel enema: Crohn's disease, coeliac disease, Whipple's disease.
- Faecal fat estimation/ERCP: pancreatic insufficiency.

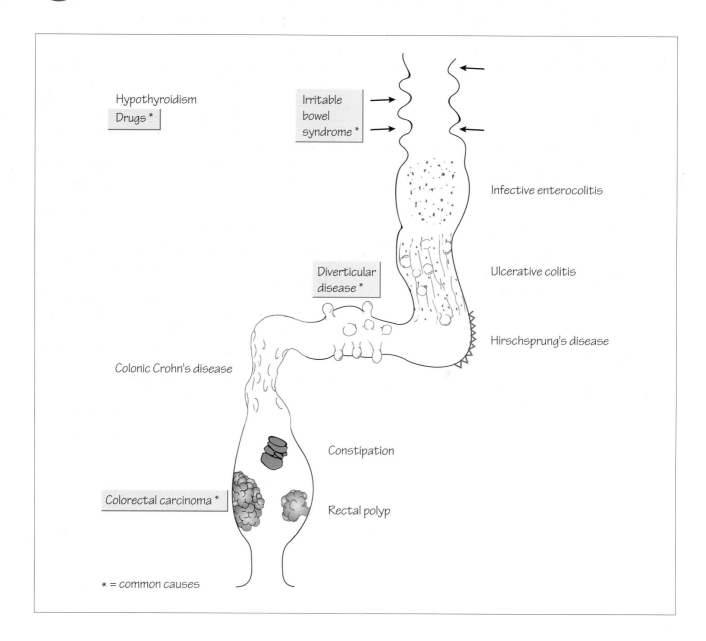

Hypothyroidism
Drugs *

Irritable bowel syndrome *

Infective enterocolitis

Diverticular disease *

Ulcerative colitis

Hirschsprung's disease

Colonic Crohn's disease

Constipation

Colorectal carcinoma *

Rectal polyp

* = common causes

Definitions

'*Normal*' *bowel habit* varies widely from person to person. Alterations in bowel habit are common manifestations of GI disease. *Constipation* is defined as infrequent or difficult evacuation of faeces and can be acute or chronic. *Absolute constipation* is defined as the inability to pass either faeces or flatus. *Diarrhoea* is an increase in the fluidity of stool.

Key points

- Acute constipation often indicates intestinal obstruction. The cardinal symptoms of obstruction are colicky abdominal pain, vomiting, constipation and distension.
- Chronic constipation may be a lifelong problem or may develop slowly in later life.
- All alterations in bowel habit that persist must be investigated for an underlying cause—colorectal neoplasms are common causes, especially in the elderly.
- IBS is a diagnosis of exclusion and should rarely be considered for new symptoms age >55

Important diagnostic features
Chronic constipation
Bowel disease

- Colon cancer: gradual onset, colicky abdominal pain, associated weight loss, anergia, anaemia, positive faecal occult bloods, abdominal mass.
- Diverticular disease: associated LIF pains, inflammatory episodes, rectal bleeding.
- Perianal pain, e.g. fissure, perianal abscess—due to spasm of the internal anal sphincter, common in children.

Adynamic bowel

- Hirschsprung's disease: constipation from birth, gross abdominal distension. Short-segment Hirschsprung's disease (involving only the lower rectum) may present in adulthood with worsening chronic constipation and megarectum/megasigmoid.
- Drugs: opiates, anticholinergics, antipsychotics, secondary to chronic laxative abuse.
- Pregnancy: due to progesterone effects on smooth muscle of bowel wall.

Key investigations

- Rectal examination: rectal cancer, rectal adenoma.
- FBC: anaemia from colon cancer, ulcerative colitis, diverticular disease.
- Stool culture: infections (remember microscopy for parasites).
- Proctoscopy/sigmoidoscopy: cancer, colitis, polyps (simple, easy, cheap and safe; performed in outpatients).
- Flexible sigmoidoscopy: cancer, polyps, colitis, infections (relatively safe, well tolerated, high sensitivity).
- Barium enema: best for tumours of proximal colon.
- Colonoscopy: colitis (extent and severity).
- Rectal biopsy (full thickness): Hirschsprung's disease.

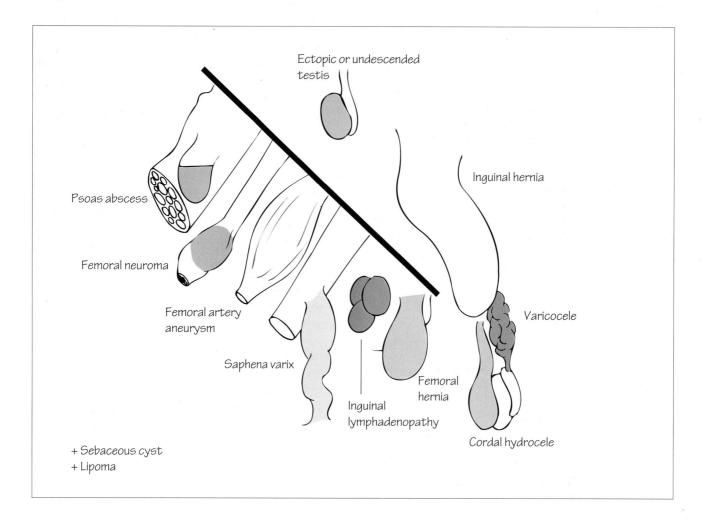

Ectopic or undescended testis

Inguinal hernia

Psoas abscess

Femoral neuroma

Femoral artery aneurysm

Saphena varix

Inguinal lymphadenopathy

Femoral hernia

Varicocele

Cordal hydrocele

+ Sebaceous cyst
+ Lipoma

Definition

Any swelling in the inguinal area or upper medial thigh.

Key points

- The groin crease does not mark the inguinal ligament in most people and is an unreliable landmark.
- Inguinal hernias are common, always start above and medial to the pubic tubercle, may be medial or lateral to it and usually emphasize the groin crease on that side.
- Femoral hernias always start below and lateral to the pubic tubercle and usually flatten the skin crease on that side.
- Femoral hernias are more common in women, are high risk and need urgent attention.
- Masses in the groin and scrotum together are inguinal hernias.
- Inguinal lymphadenopathy may be isolated or may be part of systemic lymphadenopathy. A cause should always be sought.

Important diagnostic features

The types, causes and features are listed below.

Inguinal

- Direct inguinal hernia: not controlled by pressure over internal ring, characteristically causes a 'forward' bulge in the groin, does not descend into the scrotum.
- Indirect inguinal hernia: controlled by pressure over internal ring, 'slides' through the inguinal canal, often descends into the scrotum.
- Undescended testis: often mass at the external ring or inguinal canal, associated with hypoplastic hemi-scrotum, frequently associated with indirect inguinal hernia.

- Spermatic cord: 'cordal' hydrocele, does not have a cough impulse, may be possible to define upper edge, fluctuates and transilluminates.
- Lipoma: soft, fleshy, does not transilluminate or fluctuate.

Femoral

- Femoral hernia: elderly women (mostly), may be tender and non-expansile, not reducible, groin crease often lost, high risk of strangulation and obstruction.
- Saphena varix: expansile, cough impulse, thrill on percussion of distal saphenous vein.
- Lymphadenopathy: hard, discrete nodules, often multiple or an indistinct mass.
- Femoral artery aneurysm: expansile, pulsatile, thrill and bruit may be present.
- Psoas abscess (rare): soft, fluctuant and compressible, lateral to the femoral artery, may be 'cold' abscesses caused by TB.
- Femoral neuroma (very rare): hard, smooth, moves laterally but not vertically, pressure may cause pain in the distribution of the femoral nerve.
- Hydrocele of femoral sac (very rare).

Key investigations

- FBC: causes of lymphadenopathy.
- Ultrasound: femoral aneurysm, saphena varix, psoas abscess, ectopic testicle. Also sometimes useful to identify small femoral hernias.
- CT scan: cause of psoas abscess.
- Herniography: rarely needed to confirm presence of hernia if operative indication not clear.

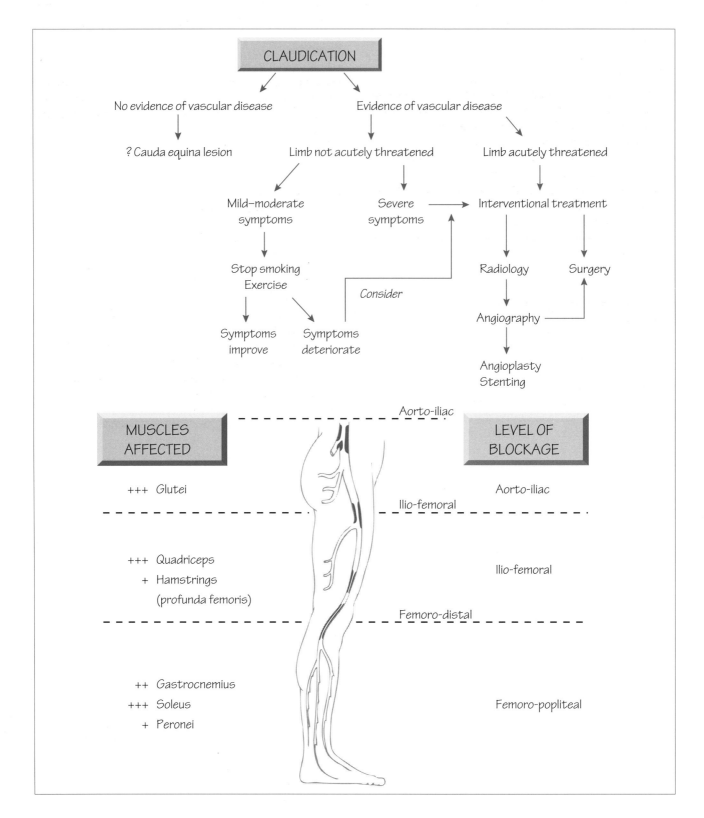

CLAUDICATION

No evidence of vascular disease

Evidence of vascular disease

? Cauda equina lesion

Limb not acutely threatened

Limb acutely threatened

Mild–moderate symptoms

Severe symptoms

Interventional treatment

Stop smoking
Exercise

Consider

Radiology

Surgery

Symptoms improve

Symptoms deteriorate

Angiography

Angioplasty
Stenting

Aorto-iliac

MUSCLES AFFECTED

LEVEL OF BLOCKAGE

+++ Glutei

Aorto-iliac

Ilio-femoral

+++ Quadriceps
 + Hamstrings
    (profunda femoris)

Ilio-femoral

Femoro-distal

 ++ Gastrocnemius
+++ Soleus
  + Peronei

Femoro-popliteal

Definition

Intermittent claudication is defined as an aching pain in the leg muscles, usually the calf, that is precipitated by walking and is relieved by rest.

Key points

- Claudication pain is always reversible and relieved by rest.
- Claudication tends to improve with time and exercise due to the opening up of new collateral supply vessels and improved muscle function.
- The site of disease is one level higher than the highest level of affected muscles.
- Most patients with claudication have associated vascular disease and investigation for occult coronary or cerebrovascular is mandatory.
- Cauda equina ischaemia caused by osteoarthritis of the spine can also cause intermittent claudication.

Differential diagnosis

Vascular

Atheroma

- Typical patient: male, over 45 years, ischaemic heart disease, smoker, diabetic, overweight.
- Aortic occlusion: buttock, thigh and possibly calf claudication, impotence in males, absent femoral pulses and below in both legs (Leriche's syndrome).
- Iliac or common femoral stenosis: thigh and calf claudication, absent/weak femoral pulses in affected limb.
- Femoro-popliteal stenosis: calf claudication only, absent popliteal and distal pulses.

Neurological

Cauda equina

Elderly patients, history of chronic back pain, pain is bilateral and in the distribution of the S1–S3 dermatomes, may be accompanied by paraesthesia in the feet and loss of ankle jerks, all peripheral pulses palpable and legs well perfused.

Key investigations

- FBC: exclude polycythaemia.
- Glucose: diabetes.
- Lipids: hyperlipidaemia.
- ABI: estimate of disease severity.
- ECG: coronary disease.
- Angiography: precise location and extent of disease, pre-procedure planning. Intravenous—easier, safer, larger volume of dye. Intra-arterial—lower dye volume, better images, higher risk of complications. Digital subtraction—best images of all. MRA – excellent images.
- Duplex scanning beginning to be used instead of angiography.

TRAUMA

Hip dislocation

Knee dislocation
Cruciate rupture
Patellar fracture

Fracture

Ankle dislocation
Collateral ligament
rupture

TUMOURS

Primary

Secondary

DEGENERATIVE

'Sciatica'
• Spondylitides
• Entrapment neuropathy

Osteoarthritis

Ruptured
Baker's cyst

Gout

INFECTION

Cellulitis

Osteomyelitis

VASCULAR

Deep vein thrombosis

Definitions

Acute leg pain is a subjective, unpleasant sensation felt somewhere in the lower limb. *Referred pain* is the perception of pain in an area remote from the site of origin of the pain, e.g. leg pain from lumbar disc herniation, knee pain from hip pathology. *Cramps* are involuntary, painful contractions of voluntary muscles. *Sciatica* is a nerve pain caused by irritation of the sciatic nerve roots characterized by lumbosacral pain radiating down the back of the thigh, lateral side of the calf and into the foot.

Key points

- May be due to pathology arising in any of the tissues of the leg.
- Constant or lasting pain suggests local pathology.
- Transient or intermittent pain suggests referred pathology.
- Systemic symptoms or upset suggests inflammation.

Important diagnostic features

Infection

- Infection of skin (cellulitis): painful, swollen, red, hot leg, associated systemic features—pyrexia, rigors, anorexia, commonly caused by *Streptococcus pyogenes*.
- Acute osteomyelitis: staphylococcal infection, affects metaphyses, acute pain, tenderness and oedema over the end of a long bone, common in children, may be history of skin infection or trauma.

Trauma

- Muscle: swollen, tender and painful, pain worse on attempted movement of the affected muscle.
- Bone: painful, tender. Swelling, deformity, discoloration, bruising and crepitus suggest fracture.

- Joints: painful, limited movement, deformity if dislocated, locking and instability with knee injury.

Degenerative

- Gout: first MTP joint (big toe), males, associated signs of joint inflammation.
- Disc herniation (sciatica): pain in distribution of one or two nerve roots, sudden onset, back pain and stiffness, lumbar scoliosis due to muscle spasm.
- Ruptured Baker's cyst: pain mostly behind the knee, previous history of knee arthritis, calf may be hot and swollen.

Tumours

Bone: deep pain, worse in morning and after exercise, overlying muscle tenderness, pathological fractures, primary (e.g. osteosarcoma, osteoclastoma) or secondary (e.g. breast, prostate, lung metastasis).

Vascular

DVT: calf pain, swelling, redness, prominent superficial veins, tender on calf compression, low-grade pyrexia.

Key investigations

- FBC: WCC in infection.
- D-Dimers: suspected DVT.
- Blood cultures: spreading cellulitis.
- Clotting: DVT.
- Plain X-ray: trauma, osteomyelitis, bone tumours, gout.
- MRI: suspected disc herniation.
- Duplex ultrasound: DVT.
- Venography: DVT where duplex not available or precise extent needed.

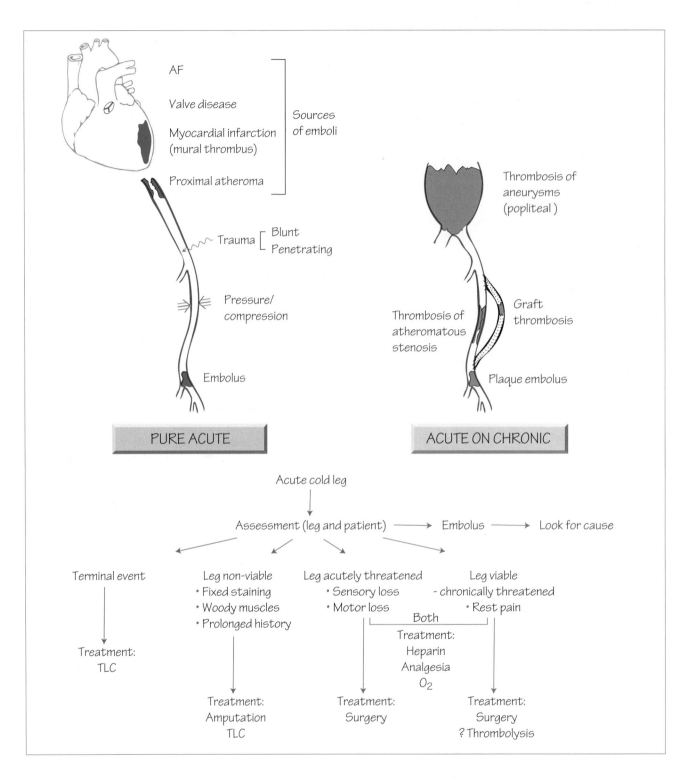

AF

Valve disease

Myocardial infarction
(mural thrombus)

Proximal atheroma

Sources
of emboli

Trauma [Blunt
Penetrating

Pressure/
compression

Embolus

PURE ACUTE

Thrombosis of
aneurysms
(popliteal)

Thrombosis of
atheromatous
stenosis

Graft
thrombosis

Plaque embolus

ACUTE ON CHRONIC

Acute cold leg

Assessment (leg and patient) ⟶ Embolus ⟶ Look for cause

Terminal event

Treatment:
TLC

Leg non-viable
• Fixed staining
• Woody muscles
• Prolonged history

Treatment:
Amputation
TLC

Leg acutely threatened
• Sensory loss
• Motor loss

Both

Treatment:
Heparin
Analgesia
O_2

Treatment:
Surgery

Leg viable
- chronically threatened
• Rest pain

Treatment:
Surgery
? Thrombolysis

Definition

The 'acute cold leg' is a clinical syndrome of the sudden onset of symptoms indicative of the presence of ischaemia sufficient to threaten the viability of the limb or part of it.

Key points

- Remember the '6 Ps' of acute ischaemia—painful, pale, paraesthetic, paralysed, pulseless, perishingly cold.
- All acute cold legs are a surgical emergency and require a prompt diagnosis.
- 80% of acute cold legs presenting as an emergency have underlying chronic vascular pathology.
- Fasciotomies should always be considered as part of treatment if a leg is being revascularized.

Important diagnostic features

Isolated arterial embolus

- Sudden-onset, severe ischaemia, no previous symptoms of vascular disease, previous history of atrial fibrillation/recent myocardial infarction, all peripheral pulses on the unaffected limb normal (suggesting no underlying peripheral vascular disease [PVD]).
- Limb usually acutely threatened due to complete occlusion with no collateral supply.
- Common sites of impaction are: popliteal bi(tri)furcation, distal superficial femoral artery (adductor canal), origin of the profunda femoris. 'Saddle' embolus at aortic bifurcation causes bilateral acute ischaemic limbs.

Trauma

- May be due to direct injury to the vessel or by secondary compression due to bone fragments or haematoma.

- Direct injuries may be due to: complete division of the vessel, distraction injury, damage and *in situ* thrombosis, foreign body, false aneurysm.

Thrombosis (*in situ*)

- Usually associated with underlying atheroma predisposing to thrombosis after minor trauma or immobility (after a fall or illness).
- May be subacute in onset, previous history of known vascular disease or intermittent claudication, associated risk factors for peripheral vascular disease, abnormal pulses in the unaffected limb.
- Paradoxically, the limb may not be as acutely threatened as in isolated arterial embolus because collateral vessels may already be present due to underlying disease.

Graft thrombosis

Often subacute in onset, limb not acutely threatened, progressive symptoms, loss of graft pulsation

Aneurysm thrombosis

- Most common site—popliteal aneurysms.
- Sudden-onset limb ischaemia, acutely threatened, may be associated embolization as well, non-pulsatile mass in popliteal fossa, many have contralateral asymptomatic popliteal aneurysm.

Key investigations

- FBC: polycythaemia.
- U+E: renal impairment, myonecrosis.
- Clotting: thrombophilia.
- ECG: atrial fibrillation, myocardial infarction, valve disease.
- Duplex scanning: graft patency, popliteal aneurysm
- Angiography: wherever possible—arterial embolism, thrombosis, underlying PVD.

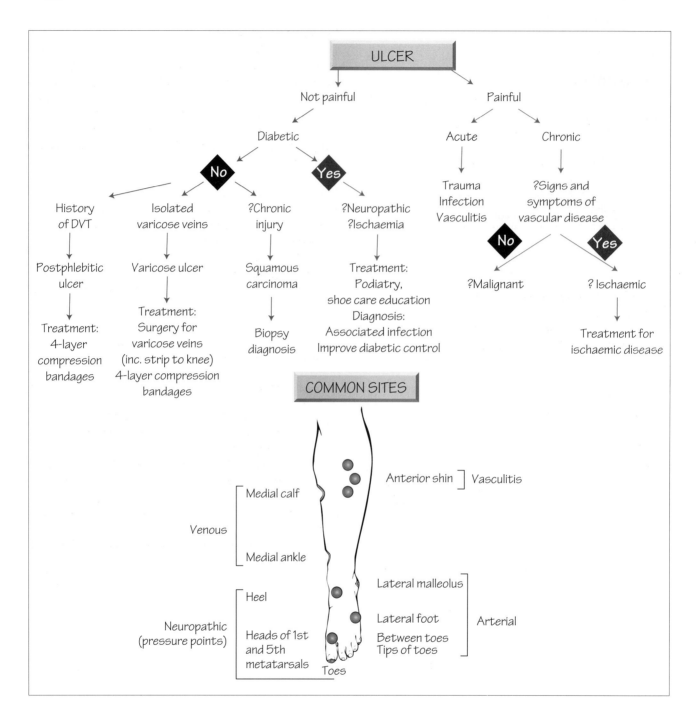

ULCER

Not painful

Painful

Diabetic

No

Yes

Acute

Chronic

History of DVT

Isolated varicose veins

?Chronic injury

?Neuropathic ?Ischaemia

Trauma Infection Vasculitis

?Signs and symptoms of vascular disease

No

Yes

Postphlebitic ulcer

Varicose ulcer

Squamous carcinoma

Treatment: Podiatry, shoe care education Diagnosis: Associated infection Improve diabetic control

?Malignant

? Ischaemic

Treatment: 4-layer compression bandages

Treatment: Surgery for varicose veins (inc. strip to knee) 4-layer compression bandages

Biopsy diagnosis

Treatment for ischaemic disease

COMMON SITES

Anterior shin] Vasculitis

Medial calf

Venous

Medial ankle

Lateral malleolus

Heel

Lateral foot

Arterial

Neuropathic (pressure points)

Heads of 1st and 5th metatarsals

Between toes Tips of toes

Toes

Definition

An *ulcer* is defined as an area of discontinuity of the surface epithelium.

Key points

- Pain suggests ischaemia or infection.
- Neuropathic ulcers occur over points of pressure and trauma.
- Marked worsening of a chronic ulcer suggests malignant change.
- The underlying cause must be treated first or the ulcer will not heal.
- Several precipitating causes may coexist (e.g. diabetes, PVD and neuropathy).
- Underlying varicose veins must be treated for venous ulcers.

Important diagnostic features

Venous ulcers

- Venous hypertension secondary to DVT or varicose veins: ulceration on the medial side of the leg, above the ankle, any size, shallow with sloping edges, bleeds after minor trauma, weeps readily, associated dermatoliposclerosis.
- If deep venous disease is suspected duplex scanning of the veins or venography is indicated.

Arterial ulcers

Occlusive arterial disease: painful ulcers, do not bleed, non-healing, lateral ankle, heel, metatarsal heads, tips of the toes, associated features of ischaemia, e.g. claudication, absent pulses, pallor. Elderly patients may present with 'blue toe' syndrome.

Diabetic ulcers

- Ischaemic: same as arterial ulcers.

- Neuropathic: deep, painless ulcers, plantar aspect of foot or toes, associated with cellulitis and deep tissue abscesses, warm foot, pulses may be present.

Malignant ulcers

- Squamous cell carcinoma: may arise *de novo* or malignant change in a chronic ulcer or burn (Marjolin's ulcer). Large ulcer, heaped up, everted edges. Lymphadenopathy—highly suspicious.
- Basal cell carcinoma: uncommon on the leg, rolled edges, pearly white.
- Malignant melanoma: lower limb is a common site, consider malignant if increase in size or pigmentation, bleeding, itching or ulceration.

Miscellaneous ulcers

- Trauma: may be caused by minor trauma. Predisposing factors are poor circulation, malnutrition or steroid treatment.
- Vasculitis (rare), e.g. rheumatoid arthritis, SLE.
- Infections (rare): syphilis, TB, tropical infections.
- Pyoderma gangrenosum: multiple necrotic ulcers over the legs that start as nodules. Seen with ulcerative colitis and Crohn's disease.

Key investigations

- FBC: infections.
- Glucose: diabetes.
- Special blood tests: TPHA (syphilis), ANCA (SLE), Rh factor.
- Ankle–brachial pressure index (ABI) measurement to exclude underlying PVD.
- Doppler ultrasound: assessment of venous disease, assessment of arterial disease (above the knee). Simple, cheap, highly sensitive, good screening test.
- Biopsy: malignancy. Melanoma—always excision biopsy. Others may be incision/'punch'.
- Venography/angiography: extent and severity of disease. Planning treatment.

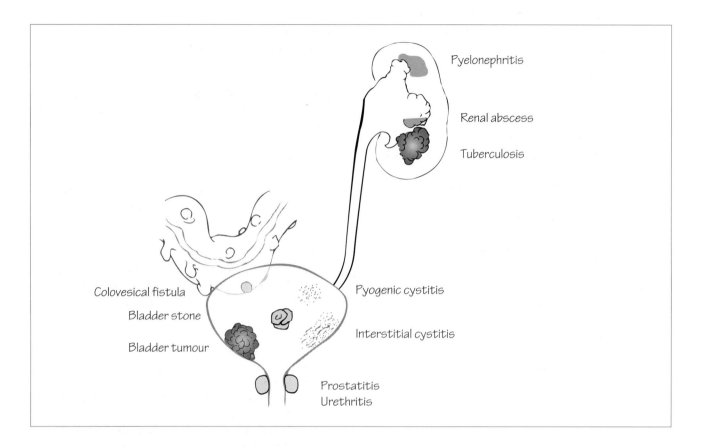

Definitions

Dysuria is defined as a pain that arises from an irritation of the urethra and is felt during micturition. *Frequency* indicates increased passage of urine during the daytime, while *nocturia* indicates increased passage of urine during the night. *Urgency* is an uncontrollable desire to micturate and may be associated with incontinence.

Key points

- UTI is the most common cause of dysuria in adults.
- Systemic upset and loin pain suggest an ascending UTI (pyelonephritis).
- Elderly men with recurrent UTIs often have an underlying problem of bladder emptying due to prostate disease.
- Recurrent infections require investigation to exclude an underlying cause.
- Pneumaturia, 'bits' in the urine and coliform infections suggest a colovesical fistula.

Important diagnostic features

Urinary tract infection

Acute pyelonephritis

Cause: Upper tract infection.

Predisposing causes **are**:
- Outflow tract obstruction.
- Vesicoureteric reflux.
- Renal or bladder calculi.
- Diabetes mellitus.
- Neuropathic bladder dysfunction.

Features: Pyrexia, rigors, flank pain, dysuria, malaise, anorexia, leucocytosis, pyuria, bacteriuria, microscopic haematuria, C&S >100 000 organisms per ml.

Acute cystitis

Causes **are**:
- Lower tract infection.
- Usually coliform bacteria.
- Because of short urethra commoner in females.
- Proteus infections may indicate stone disease.

Features: Dysuria, frequency, urgency, suprapubic pain, low back pain, incontinence and microscopic haematuria.

Urethritis

Causes **are**:
- Sexually transmitted diseases.
- May be gonococcal, chlamydial or mycoplasmal.

Features: Dysuria and meatal pruritus, occurs 3–10 days after sexual contact, yellowish purulent urethral discharge suggests Gonococcus, thin mucoid discharge suggests *Chlamydia*.

Other causes of dysuria

Urethral syndrome

A condition characterized by frequency, urgency and dysuria in women with urine cultures showing no growth or low bacterial counts.

Vaginitis

Condition characterized by dysuria, pruritus and vaginal discharge. Urine cultures are negative, but vaginal cultures often reveal *Trichomonas vaginalis*, *Candida albicans* or *Haemophilus vaginalis*.

Bladder tumours

- Uncommon cause of dysuria, haematuria, sterile pyuria (no growth on MSU).
- Ultrasound: possible pyelonephritis/renal abscess, may show predisposing structural abnormality.
- DMSA scan: assesses renal function where renal damage suspected from recurrent sepsis.

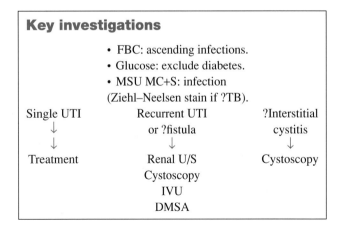

Key investigations

- FBC: ascending infections.
- Glucose: exclude diabetes.
- MSU MC+S: infection (Ziehl–Neelsen stain if ?TB).

Single UTI	Recurrent UTI or ?fistula	?Interstitial cystitis
↓	↓	↓
↓		
Treatment	Renal U/S Cystoscopy IVU DMSA	Cystoscopy

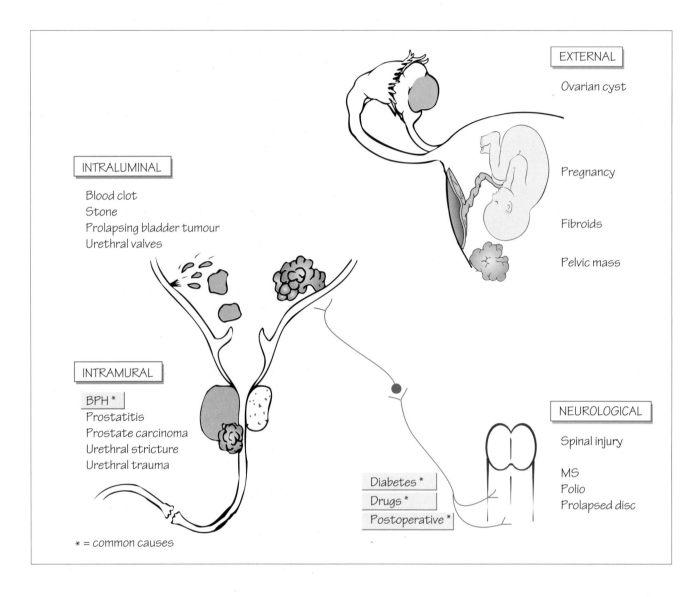

INTRALUMINAL

Blood clot
Stone
Prolapsing bladder tumour
Urethral valves

INTRAMURAL

BPH *
Prostatitis
Prostate carcinoma
Urethral stricture
Urethral trauma

* = common causes

EXTERNAL

Ovarian cyst

Pregnancy

Fibroids

Pelvic mass

NEUROLOGICAL

Spinal injury

MS
Polio
Prolapsed disc

Diabetes *
Drugs *
Postoperative *

Definitions

Urinary retention is defined as an inability to micturate. *Acute urinary retention* is the sudden inability to micturate in the presence of a painful bladder. *Chronic urinary retention* is the presence of an enlarged, full, painless bladder with or without difficulty in micturition. *Overflow incontinence* is an uncontrollable leakage and dribbling of urine from the urethra in the presence of a full bladder.

Key points

- Acute retention is characterized by pain, sensation of bladder fullness and a mildly distended bladder.
- Remember common causes:
  children—abdominal pain, drugs
  young—postoperative, drugs, acute UTI, trauma, haematuria
  elderly—acute on chronic retention with BPH, tumours, postoperative.
- **Chronic retention** is characterized by symptoms of bladder irritation (frequency, dysuria, small volume), or painless, marked distension, overflow incontinence (often associated with secondary UTI).
- Remember common causes:
  children—congenital abnormalities
  young—trauma, postoperative
  elderly—BPH, strictures, prostatic carcinoma.
- **Neurogenic retention**.
- Upper motor neurone causes produce chronic retention with reflex incontinence.
- Lower motor neurone causes produce chronic retention with overflow incontinence.
- Urinary retention is uncommon in young adults and almost always requires investigation to exclude underlying cause.
- Retention is common in elderly men—often due to prostate pathology.

Differential diagnosis
Mechanical
In the lumen of the urethra
- Congenital valves (rare): neonates, males, recurrent UTIs.
- Foreign body (rare).
- Stones (rare): acute pain in penis and glans.
- Tumour (rare): TCC or squamous cell carcinoma, history of haematuria, working in dye or rubber industry.

In the wall of the urethra
- BPH: frequency, nocturia, hesitancy, poor stream, dribbling, urgency.
- Tumour: as above.
- Stricture: history of trauma or serious infection, gradual onset of poor stream.
- Trauma: blood at meatus.

Outside the wall of the urethra
- Pregnancy.
- Fibroids: palpable, bulky uterus, menorrhagia, dysmenorrhoea.
- Ovarian cyst: mobile iliac fossa mass.
- Faecal impaction: spurious diarrhoea.

Neurological
- Postoperative: pain, drugs, pelvic nerve disturbance.
- Spinal cord injuries: acute phase is lower motor neurone type, late phase is upper motor neurone type.
- Drugs: narcotics, anticholinergics, antihistamines, antipsychotics.
- Diabetes: progressive lower motor neurone pattern.
- Idiopathic: detrusor sphincter dyssynergia, ?bladder neurone degeneration.

Key investigations

- U+E: renal function.
- MSU MC+S: associated infection, include cytology where tumour suspected.
- Cystography: urethral valves, strictures.
- IVU: renal/bladder stones.
- Urodynamics: allows identification and assessment of neurological problems, assesses BPH.
- Cystoscopy.

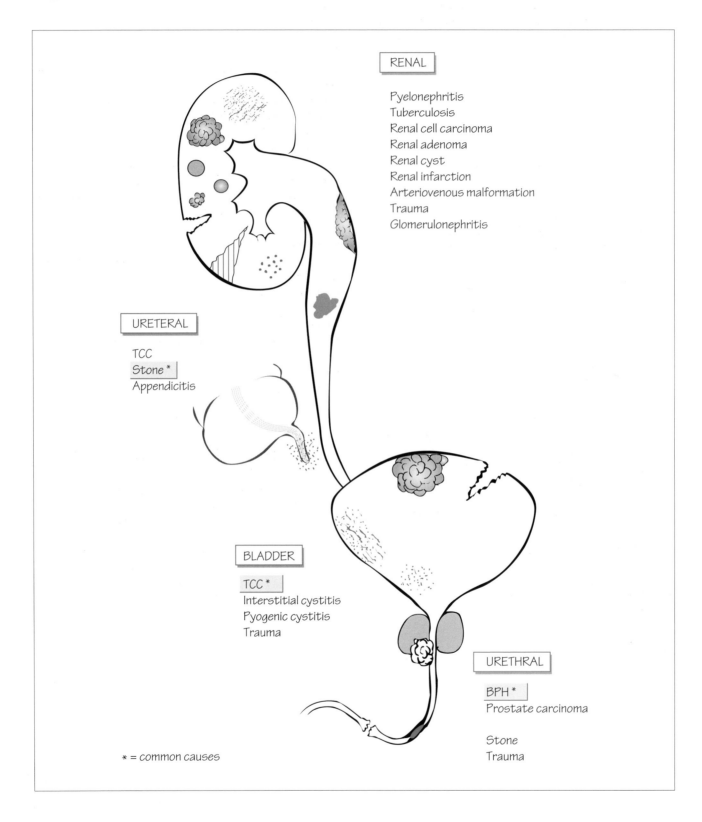

RENAL

Pyelonephritis
Tuberculosis
Renal cell carcinoma
Renal adenoma
Renal cyst
Renal infarction
Arteriovenous malformation
Trauma
Glomerulonephritis

URETERAL

TCC
Stone *
Appendicitis

BLADDER

TCC *
Interstitial cystitis
Pyogenic cystitis
Trauma

URETHRAL

BPH *
Prostate carcinoma

Stone
Trauma

* = common causes

Definitions

Haematuria is the passage of blood in the urine. *Frank haematuria* is the presence of blood on macroscopic examination, while *microscopic haematuria* indicates that RBCs are only seen on microscopy. *Haemoglobinuria* is defined as the presence of free Hb in the urine.

Key points

• Haematuria always requires investigation to exclude an underlying cause.
• Initial haematuria (blood on commencing urination) suggests a urethral cause.
• Terminal haematuria (blood after passing urine) suggests a bladder base or prostatic cause.
• Ribbon clots suggest a pelvi-ureteric cause.
• Renal bleeding can mimic colic due to clots passing down the ureter.

Important diagnostic features

Kidney

• Trauma: mild to moderate trauma commonly causes renal bleeding, severe injuries may not bleed (avulsed kidney—complete disruption).
• Tumours: may be profuse or intermittent.
• Renal cell carcinoma: associated mass, loin pain, clot colic or fever, occasional polycythaemia, hypercalcaemia and hypertension.
• TCC: characteristically painless, intermittent haematuria.
• Calculus: severe loin/groin pain, gross or microscopic, associated infection.
• Glomerulonephritis: usually microscopic, associated systemic disease (e.g. SLE).
• Pyelonephritis (rare).
• Renal tuberculosis (rare): sterile pyuria, weight loss, anorexia, PUO, increased frequency of micturition day and night.
• Polycystic disease (rare): palpable kidneys, hypertension, chronic renal failure.
• Renal arteriovenous malformation or simple cyst (very rare): painless, no other symptoms.
• Renal infarction (very rare): may be caused by an arterial embolus, painful tender kidney.

Ureter

• Calculus: severe loin/groin pain, gross or microscopic, associated infection.
• TCC: see below.

Bladder

• Calculus: sudden cessation of micturition, pain in perineum and tip of penis.
• TCC: characteristically painless, intermittent haematuria, history of work in rubber or dye industries.
• Acute cystitis: suprapubic pain, dysuria, frequency and bacteriuria.
• Interstitial cystitis (rare): may be autoimmune, drug or radiation induced, frequency and dysuria common.
• Schistosomiasis (very rare): history of foreign travel, especially North Africa.

Prostate

• BPH: painless haematuria, associated obstructive symptoms, recurrent UTI.
• Carcinoma (rare).

Urethra

• Trauma: blood at meatus, history of direct blow to perineum, acute retention.
• Calculus (rare).
• Urethritis (rare).

Key investigations

• FBC: infection, chronic blood loss. 'Rouleaux' suggest glomerulonephritis.
• Clotting: exclude underlying bleeding cause.
• U+E: renal function.
• MSU MC+S: infection, parasites.

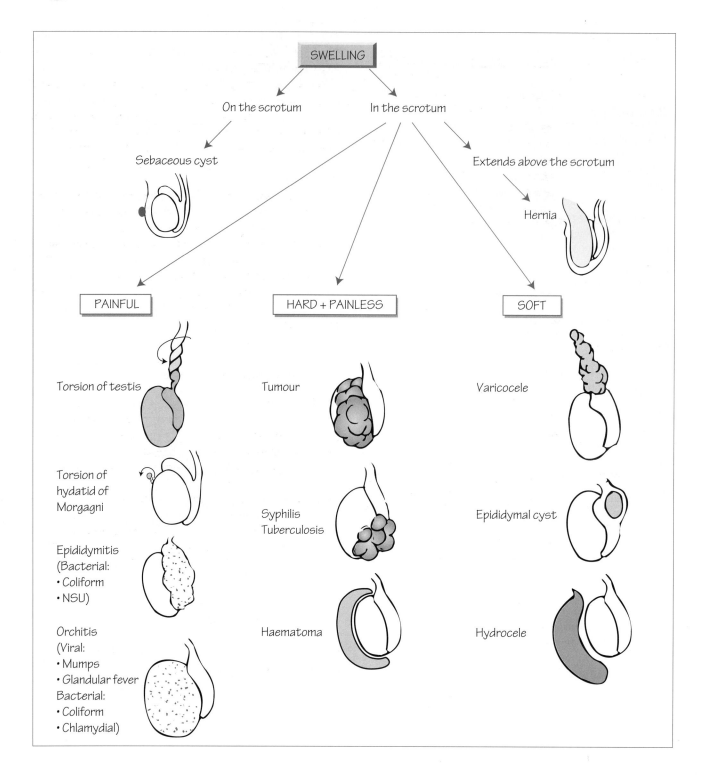

Definition

Any swelling in or on the scrotum or its contents.

Key points

- Always evaluate scrotal swellings for extension to the groin. If present they are almost always inguinoscrotal hernias.
- Torsion is most common in adolescence and in the early twenties. Whenever the diagnosis is suspected, urgent assessment and usually surgery are required.
- Young adult men: tumours, trauma and acute infections are common.
- Old men: hydrocele and hernia are common.

Differential diagnosis

The causes and features are listed below.

Scrotum

- Sebaceous cyst: attached to the skin, just fluctuant, does not transilluminate.
- Infantile scrotal oedema: acute idiopathic scrotal swelling, hot, tender, bright red, testicle less tender than in torsion, most common in young boys.

Testis

Painful conditions

- Orchitis: confined to testis, young men.
- Epididymo-orchitis: painful and swollen, epididymis more than testis, associated erythema of scrotum, fever and pyuria, unusual below the age of 25 years, pain relieved by elevating the testis.
- Torsion of the testis: rapid onset, pubertal males, often high investment of tunica vaginalis on the cord —'bellclapper testis', testis may lie high and transversely in the scrotum, 'knot' in the cord may be felt.
- Torsion of appendix testis: mimics full torsion, early signs are a lump at the upper pole of the testis and a blue spot on transillumination, later the whole testis becomes swollen, may require explorative surgery to exclude full torsion.

Hard conditions

- Testicular tumour: painless swelling, younger adult men (20–50 years), may have lax secondary hydrocele, associated abdominal lymphadenopathy.
- Haematocele: firm, does not transilluminate, testis cannot usually be felt, history of trauma.
- Syphilitic gummata—firm, rubbery, usually associated with other features of secondary syphilis. TB—uncommon outside developing world, usually associated with miliary disease.

Soft conditions

- Hydrocele: soft, fluctuant, transilluminates brilliantly, testis may be difficult to feel, new onset or rapidly recurrent hydrocele suggests an underlying testicular cause.
- Epididymal cyst: separate and behind the testis, transilluminates well, may be quite large.
- Varicocele: a collection of dilated and tortuous veins in the spermatic cord—'bag of worms' on examination, more common on the left, associated with a dragging sensation, occasional haematospermia.

Key investigations

- FBC: infection.
- Ultrasound: painless, non-invasive imaging of testicle. Allows underlying pathology to be excluded in hydrocele. High sensitivity and specificity for tumours.
- Doppler ultrasound: may confirm presence of blood flow where torsion is thought unlikely.
- CT scan: staging for testicular tumours.
- Surgery: may be the only way to confirm or exclude torsion in a high-risk group. Should not be delayed for any other investigation if required.

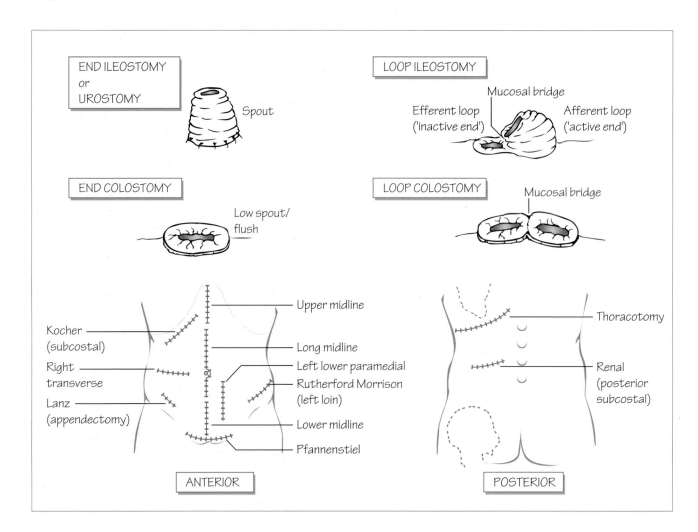

END ILEOSTOMY or UROSTOMY

Spout

LOOP ILEOSTOMY

Mucosal bridge

Efferent loop ('inactive end')

Afferent loop ('active end')

END COLOSTOMY

Low spout/flush

LOOP COLOSTOMY

Mucosal bridge

Kocher (subcostal)

Right transverse

Lanz (appendectomy)

Upper midline

Long midline

Left lower paramedial

Rutherford Morrison (left loin)

Lower midline

Pfannenstiel

ANTERIOR

Thoracotomy

Renal (posterior subcostal)

POSTERIOR

Definitions

A *stoma* is an opening from a hollow viscus connecting it to the skin surface. An *ileostomy* is an opening in the small intestine. A *colostomy* is an opening in the large intestine. A *urostomy* is an external opening in the urinary tract. The most common form is a short length of ileum formed into a stoma and connected to the urinary tract (ureters) to act as a conduit for urine (ileal conduit). A *laparotomy* is any incision in the abdominal wall.

Key points

- Ileostomies and urostomies are usually spouted to reduce the risk of the output causing irritation of the surrounding skin.
- Colostomies are usually flush to the skin.
- Don't assume what type of stoma is present by its location.

Complications of stomas

- Necrosis—acute early complication due to compromised blood supply—appears black or dark purple. Rx—re-operation to remake the stoma.
- Stenosis—narrowing of stoma or cutaneous orifice usually due to small skin defect or chronic ischaemia of stoma. Rx—dilatation by probe dilators or refashioning of stoma by surgery.
- Retraction—spout reduced/absent or stoma indrawn into abdominal wall—usually due to tension on the bowel used. Rx—convex stoma appliances, refashioning of stoma by surgery.
- Prolapse—excessive spout length—due to loose skin defect or chronic effect of bowel peristalsis. More common in loop stomas especially loop colostomies. Rx—stoma appliance change or refashioning of stoma.
- Herniation—presence of bowel in the subcutaneous tissues. Usually due to an oversized opening in the abdominal muscles wall. Most common stoma complication long term. Often causes problems with stoma appliance adherence. Rx—repair hernia, resiting stoma.
- Peristomal dermatitis—due to contents spilling onto peristomal skin or trauma of appliance changes. Rx—better stoma care, change of appliance, topical anti-inflammatories.
- Fluid and electrolyte imbalances—usually only a problem in ileostomies (especially early after formation, if high in the small bowel or associated gastroenteritis). Caused by excessive wash-out of electrolyte rich fluid. Rx—control of high output (dietary modifications, use of anti-diarrhoeals, temporary use of isotonic oral fluids), intravenous fluid replacement if severe.

Features to recognize a stoma

- Fully spouted stomas are almost always formed from ileum. They may be an ileostomy or a urostomy.
- Spouted stomas with two lumens are always loop ileostomies. Look carefully to identify a second lumen as it may not be obvious.
- Flush stomas are usually colostomies.
- Although ileostomies are often placed in the right lower abdomen and colostomies are placed in the left lower abdomen, location is never a good indication of what type of stoma is present.
- Stoma appliance contents—ileostomies usually produce semi-liquid green–brown output, colostomies usually produce solid/semi-solid faecal output. Beware—this is often unreliable in disease processes or soon after formation where the outputs may be similar. Urostomies drain clear fluid.

Siting and care of a stoma

- Electively formed stomas should be sited pre-operatively by the stoma specialist. Features to take into account are—abdominal size and shape, skin folds/creases (avoid), previous scars(avoid), level of the belt or dress line (place stomas above OR below but not ON), manual dexterity and visual impairment of patient.
- Stoma appliances are extremely varied—they may be one or two piece (separate bag and adherent flange), flat or convex, drainable or sealed, with or without odour filters.

Abdominal and thoracic incisions

- Vertical incisions are usually non-muscle splitting but traverse several or many myotomes/dermatomes.
- Tranverse incisions are usually muscle splitting but are placed to lie in one or two myotomes/dermatomes.
- Midline vertical incisions can easily be extended to improve access to all parts of the abdomen but are often larger than transverse incisions placed over the area to be operated on.
- Midline vertical incisions tend to be used where the extent or type of surgery is large or uncertain.
- Transverse incisions tend to have a lower risk of wound hernia formation.
- Thoracotomy incisions are placed between ribs and are muscle splitting.
- Thoracotomy incisions may involve division or disarticulation of the rib above or below the incision.

PRE-OPERATIVE ASSESSMENT

- Performed by anaesthetist
- Condition of patient (ASA 1–V)
- Type of surgery (minor, intermediate, major)
- Urgency of procedure (emergency, elective)

GENERAL ANAESTHESIA

Induction	Anaesthesia	Recovery

Induce loss of consciousness

Balanced anaesthesia

Maintain anaesthesia

Provide analgesia

Muscle relaxation

Maintain physiology

'Wake up' patient

Continue monitoring post-op

Pain relief

Pharmacological
– MEAC
– PCA
Physical
Psychological

Maintain airway
- Laryngeal mask
- E.T. tube
- Ventilation

Good i.v. access

Monitor

ECG
BP 120/80
O$_2$ sat 99%
(CVP)

Urinary output

Definitions

Anaesthesia ($\alpha\nu\alpha\iota\sigma\theta\epsilon\sigma\iota\alpha$ = without perception): 1. a partial or complete loss of all forms of sensation caused by pathology in the nervous system, 2. a technique using drugs (inhalational, intravenous or local) that renders the whole or part of the organism insensible for variable periods of time. *Analgesia*: the loss of pain sensation. *Hypnotic agent*: a sleep-inducing drug. *Muscle relaxant*: a drug that reduces muscle tension by affecting the nerves to muscles or the myoneuronal junction (e.g curare, succinylcholine). *Sedation*: the production of a calm and restful state by the administration of a drug.

Pre-operative assessment

Prior to an operation the anaesthetist will assess the patient and devise a plan for anaesthesia based on the following:

• The condition of the patient (ASA classification) determined by:
  – history
  – physical examination
  – selective investigations
• The complexity of the surgery to be performed.
• The urgency of the procedure (emergency or elective).

Class	ASA Preoperative physical status classification
Class I	Fit and healthy
Class II	Mild systemic disease
Class III	Severe systemic disease that is not incapacitating
Class IV	Incapacitating systemic disease that is constantly life-threatening
Class V	Moribund—not expected to survive > 24 h without surgery

ASA = American Society of Anesthesiologists

General anaesthesia

Aims and technique

• To induce a loss of consciousness using hypnotic drugs which may administered intravenously (e.g. propofol) or by inhalation (e.g. sevoflurane).
• To provide adequate operating conditions for the duration of the surgical procedure using *balanced anaesthesia* i.e. a combination of hypnotic drugs to maintain anaesthesia (e.g. propofol, sevoflurane), analgesics for pain (e.g. opiates, NSAIDS) and, if indicated, muscle relaxants (e.g. suxamethonium, tubocurarine) or regional anaesthesia.
• To maintain essential physiological function by:
  – providing a clear airway (laryngeal mask airway or tracheal tube ± intermittent positive pressure ventilation)
  – maintaining good vascular access (large bore i.v. cannula ± central venous catheter ± arterial cannula)
  – monitoring vital functions:
    • pulse oximetry (functional arterial O_2 saturation in %)
    • capnography (expired respiratory gas CO_2 level)
    • arterial blood pressure (non-invasive {sphigmomanometer} or invasive {arterial cannula}techniques)
    • temperature
    • ECG
    • ± hourly urinary output, CVP
    • (rarely: pulmonary arterial pressure, pulmonary capillary wedge pressure and cardiac output measure via a Swan–Ganz catheter).
• To awaken the patient safely at the end of the procedure.

Anaesthesia—regional

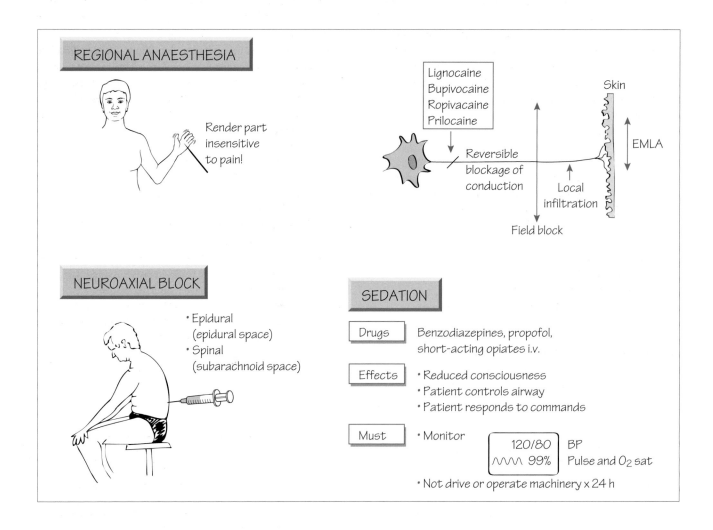

REGIONAL ANAESTHESIA

Render part insensitive to pain!

Lignocaine
Bupivocaine
Ropivacaine
Prilocaine

Skin

EMLA

Reversible blockage of conduction

Local infiltration

Field block

NEUROAXIAL BLOCK

• Epidural (epidural space)
• Spinal (subarachnoid space)

SEDATION

Drugs — Benzodiazepines, propofol, short-acting opiates i.v.

Effects
• Reduced consciousness
• Patient controls airway
• Patient responds to commands

Must
• Monitor

120/80 — BP
99% — Pulse and O_2 sat

• Not drive or operate machinery x 24 h

Regional anaesthesia

Aims and technique

• To render an area of the body completely insensitive to pain.
• Local anaesthetic agents (LA) prevent pain by causing a reversible blockof conduction along nerve axons. Addition of a vasoconstrictor (e.g. adrenaline) reduces systemic absorption allowing more LA to be given and prolonging its duration of action.

	Dose-mg/kg (+ adrenaline)	Possible systemic toxicity of local anaesthetic agents
Lignocaine	3 (7)	CNS—headache, drowsiness,
Bupivacaine	2 (2)	confusion, visual disturbance,
Ropivacaine	2 (2)	headache, nausea, vomiting
Prilocaine	4 (7)	RS—respiratory arrest
		CVS—altered BP, arrhythmias

Regional anaesthetic techniques

• Topical administration of local anaesthetic (LA is placed on the skin—e.g. EMLA® (**E**utetic **M**ixture of **L**ocal **A**naesthetic) cream prior to venepuncture).
• Local infiltration of LA (subcutaneous infiltration around the immediate surrounding area—e.g. used for excision of skin lesions).
• Field block (subcutaneous infiltration of LA around an operative field to render the whole operative field anaesthetic —e.g. used for inguinal hernia repair).
• Local blocks of specific peripheral nerves (e.g. sciatic nerve block, ring block of fingers/toes, intercostals nerve block).
• Local blocks of specific plexuses (e.g. brachial plexus block for upper limb surgery, coeliac plexus block for cancer pain).
• Intravenous blocks (e.g. Bier's block of the upper limb—a short acting LA is injected via a cannula into an exsanguinated arm to which a tourniquet has been applied).

- Neuroaxial block:
  – epidural anaesthesia—local anaesthetic is injected as a bolus or via a small catheter into the epidural space. It can be used as the sole anaesthetic for surgery below the waistline, especially useful in obstetrics, or as an adjunct to general anaesthesia.
  – spinal anaesthesia—local anaesthetic is injected into the CSF in the subarachnoid space. The extent and duration of anaesthesia depend on the position of the patient, the specific gravity of the LA and the level of injection (usually lumbar spine level).

Sedation

Many minimally invasive procedures (e.g. colonoscopy) are performed under sedation only. Sedation is induced by administrating a drug or combination of drugs (e.g. benzdiazepines [*midazolam*], propofol ± short-acting opioids [*pethedine, fentanyl*]. During sedation the patient:

- has a reduced level of consciousness
- is free from anxiety
- is able to protect the airway
- is able to respond to verbal commands
- must be monitored (vital signs, pulse oximeter, ECG, level of consciousness)
- may be given an antagonist (*naloxone, flumazenil*) if oversedated (e.g. signs of respiratory depression).

After sedation the patient must be monitored until fully alert and must not drive or operate machinery for 24 hours.

Postoperative pain control

- Pain is a complex symptom with physiological (*nociception* = neural detection of pain) and psychological (*anxiety, depression*) aspects and is an inevitable consequence of surgery. *Neuopathic* pain is caused by damage to the nerve pathways.
- Methods of analgesia:
  - Pharmacological—drugs must achieve **M**inimum **E**ffective **A**nalgesic Concentration and may be administered :
    - Oral
    - Rectal
    - Transdermal
    - Subcutaneous
    - Intramuscular
    - i.v. infusion
    - i.v. bolus
    - i.v. patient controlled
    - epidural
    - nerve blocks
  - Physical
    - Splinting, immobilization and traction
    - Physiotherapy
    - Transcutaneous electrical nerve stimulation (TENS)
  - Psychological methods
- All hospitals should have an *acute pain team* to improve postoperative analgesia
- Patient controlled analgesia (PCA) is a system whereby the patient can self-administer parenteral opioids to achieve pain relief. The system requires careful patient selection and monitoring but is a very effective method of pain relief.

Type of analgesic	Effects and mode of action	Side-effects
Non-opioid		
Paracetemol	• Analgesic and antipyretic. Inhibits prostaglandin production centrally	Hepatic necrosis in large doses
NSAID	• Analgesic, anti-inflammatory, antipyretic, antiplatelet	Gastric irritation and ulceration,
Salicylates	Inhibit COX enzyme in peripheral tissue thus reducing prostaglandin	altered haemostasis, CNS toxicity,
Acetic acids	induced inflammation and nocioceptor stimulation. COX 2 inhibitors	renal impairment, asthma
Propionic acids	do not impair beneficial COX 1 effects (e.g. cytoprotection)	
Opioid		
Morphine	• Act on opioid receptors μ, κ, δ.	N&V, constipation, drowsiness,
Diamorphine	Stimulation causes:	RD, tolerance, dependence
Pethidine	μ—analgesia, RD, euphoria, dependence, N&V	
Fentanyl	κ—spinal analgesia, sedation, miosiss	
Codeine	δ—analgesia, RD, euphoria, constipation	
Tramadol		
Adjuvant		
Antidepressants	• Analgesia (but not primary action of drug)	
Anticonvulsants	Used mostly in chronic pain states	

NSAID = Non-steroidal anti-inflammatory; COX = cyclo-oxygenase; RD = respiratory depression; N&V = nausea and vomiting.

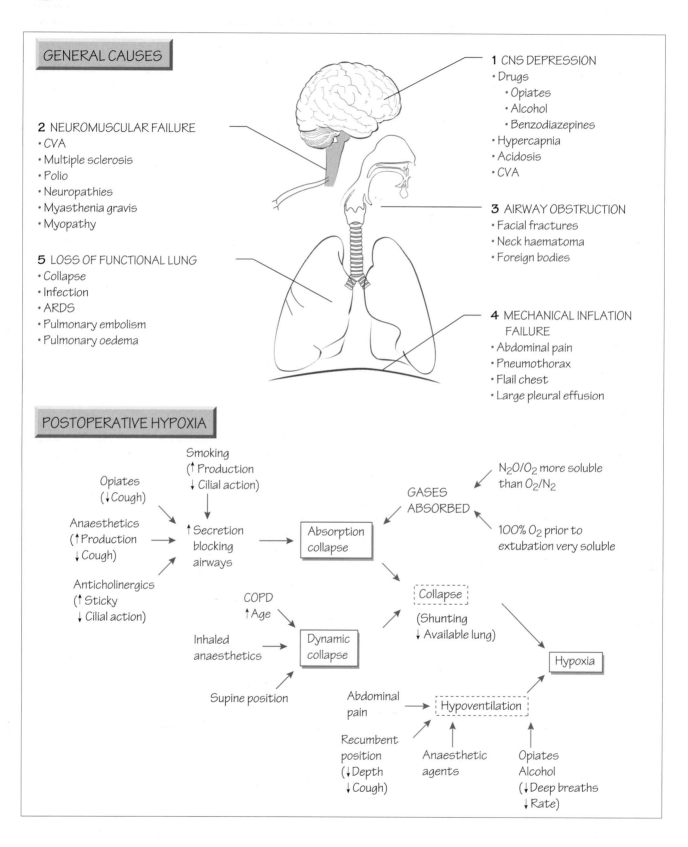

GENERAL CAUSES

2 NEUROMUSCULAR FAILURE
- CVA
- Multiple sclerosis
- Polio
- Neuropathies
- Myasthenia gravis
- Myopathy

5 LOSS OF FUNCTIONAL LUNG
- Collapse
- Infection
- ARDS
- Pulmonary embolism
- Pulmonary oedema

1 CNS DEPRESSION
- Drugs
  - Opiates
  - Alcohol
  - Benzodiazepines
- Hypercapnia
- Acidosis
- CVA

3 AIRWAY OBSTRUCTION
- Facial fractures
- Neck haematoma
- Foreign bodies

4 MECHANICAL INFLATION FAILURE
- Abdominal pain
- Pneumothorax
- Flail chest
- Large pleural effusion

POSTOPERATIVE HYPOXIA

Opiates (↓Cough)

Smoking (↑Production ↓Cilial action)

Anaesthetics (↑Production ↓Cough)

Anticholinergics (↑Sticky ↓Cilial action)

→ ↑Secretion blocking airways → Absorption collapse

GASES ABSORBED

N_2O/O_2 more soluble than O_2/N_2

100% O_2 prior to extubation very soluble

COPD ↑Age

Inhaled anaesthetics → Dynamic collapse

Supine position

Collapse (Shunting ↓Available lung)

Abdominal pain → Hypoventilation

Recumbent position (↓Depth ↓Cough)

Anaesthetic agents

Opiates Alcohol (↓Deep breaths ↓Rate)

Hypoxia

Definitions

Hypoxia is defined as a lack of O_2 (usually meaning lack of O_2 delivery to tissues or cells). *Hypoxaemia* is a lack of O_2 in arterial blood. *Apnoea* means cessation of breathing in expiration.

Common causes

Postoperative causes

- CNS depression, e.g. post-anaesthesia.
- Airway obstruction, e.g. aspiration of blood or vomit.
- Poor ventilation, e.g. abdominal pain, mechanical disruption to ventilation.
- Loss of functioning lung, e.g. ventilation–perfusion mismatch (pulmonary embolism, pneumothorax, collapse/consolidation).

General causes

- CNS depression, e.g. opiates, CVA, head injury.
- Airway obstruction, e.g. facial fractures, aspiration of blood or vomit, thyroid disease or cervical malignancy.
- Poor ventilation, e.g. pleural effusions, neuromuscular failure.
- Loss of functioning lung, e.g. ventilation–perfusion mismatch (pulmonary embolism, pneumothorax, collapse/consolidation), right to left pulmonary shunt.

Key points

- 80% of patients following upper abdominal surgery are hypoxic during the first 48 h postoperatively. Have a high index of suspicion and treat prophylactically.
- Adequate analgesia is more important than the sedative effects of opiates—ensure good analgesia in all postoperative patients.
- Ensure the dynamics of respiration are adequate—upright position, abdominal support, humidified O_2.
- Acutely confused (elderly) patients on a surgical ward are hypoxic until proven otherwise.
- Pulse oximetry saturations of less than 85% equate to an arterial $P_{O_2} < 8$ kPa and are unreliable in patients with poor peripheral perfusion.

Analgesia in postoperative patients

- Opiates: powerful, highly effective if given by correct route (e.g. PCA) but antitussive, sedative only in overdose.

- Epidural: excellent for upper abdominal/thoracic surgery, can cause hypotension by relative hypovolaemia.

Clinical features

In the unconscious patient

- Central cyanosis.
- Abnormal respirations.
- Hypotension.

In the conscious patient

- Central cyanosis.
- Anxiety, restlessness and confusion.
- Tachypnoea.
- Tachycardia, dysrhythmias (AF) and hypotension.

Key investigations

- Pulse oximetry saturations: give a guide to arterial oxygenation.
- Arterial blood gases (P_{CO_2} P_{O_2} pH base excess): respiratory acidosis, metabolic acidosis later.
- Chest X-ray: ?collapse/pneumothorax/consolidation.
- ECG: AF.

Essential management

- **Airway** control.
- Triple airway manoeuvre, suction secretions, clear oropharynx.
- Consider endotracheal intubation in CNS depression/exhausted patients (rising P_{CO_2}), neuromuscular failure.
- Consider surgical airway (cricothyroidotomy/mini-tracheostomy) in facial trauma, upper airway obstruction.
- **Breathing**.
- Position patient—upright.
- Adequate analgesia.
- Supplemental O_2—mask/bag/ventilation.
- Support respiratory physiology—physiotherapy, humidified gases, encouraging coughing, bronchodilators.
- **Circulatory** support.
- Maintain cardiac output.
- Ensure adequate fluid resuscitation.
- **Determine** and treat the cause.

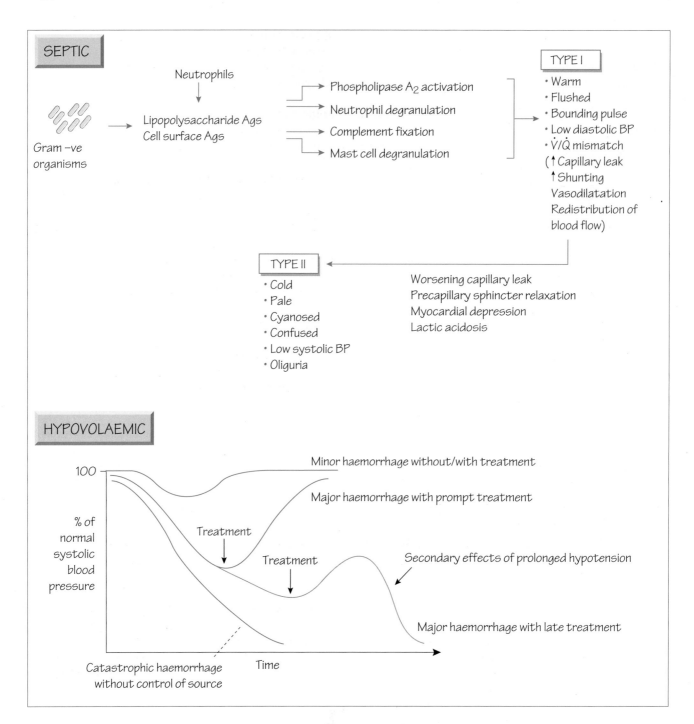

Definition

Shock is defined as a state of acute inadequate or inappropriate tissue perfusion resulting in generalized cellular hypoxia and dysfunction.

Key points

- Identify the cause early and begin treatment quickly.
- Shock in surgical patients is often overlooked—unwell, confused, restless patients may well be shocked.
- Unless a cardiogenic cause is obvious, treat shock with urgent fluid resuscitation.
- Worsening clinical status despite adequate volume replacement suggests the need for intensive care.

Common causes

Hypovolaemic

- Blood loss (ruptured abdominal aortic aneurysm, upper GI bleed, multiple fractures, etc.).
- Plasma loss (burns, pancreatitis).
- Extracellular fluid losses (vomiting, diarrhoea, intestinal fistula).

Cardiogenic

- Myocardial infarction.
- Dysrhythmias (AF, VT, AFlutter).
- Pulmonary embolus.
- Cardiac tamponade.
- Valvular heart disease

Septic

Gram −ve or, less often, Gram +ve infections.

Anaphylactic/distributive

Release of vasoactive substances when a sensitized individual is exposed to the appropriate antigen.

Clinical features

Hypovolaemic and cardiogenic

- Pallor, coldness, sweating and restlessness.
- Tachycardia, weak pulse, low BP and oliguria.

Septic

- Initially warm, flushed skin and bounding pulse.
- Later confusion and low output picture.

Investigations and assessment

- Monitor pulse, BP, temperature, respiratory rate and urinary output.
- Establish good i.v. access and set up CVP line (possibly Swan–Ganz catheter as well).
- ECG, cardiac enzymes, echocardiography.
- Hb, Hct, U+E, creatinine.
- Group and crossmatch blood: haemorrhage.
- Blood cultures: sepsis.
- Arterial blood gases.

Complications

- 'SIRS' (see p. 76) may ensue if shock not corrected.
- Acute renal failure (acute tubular necrosis).
- Hepatic failure.
- Stress ulceration.

Essential management

- **Airway and breathing**: give 100% O_2, sit up, consider ventilatory support if necessary.
- **Circulation**: ensure good i.v. access, urinary catheter, monitor cardiac rate and rhythm.

Anaphylactic
- i.v. fluids.
- i.v. adrenaline.
- i.v. antihistamines.
- i.v. hydrocortisone.

Cardiogenic
- Optimize rate and rhythm (e.g. cardioversion, drugs).
- Optimize preload (e.g. adequate volume, diuretics).
- Optimize afterload (e.g. vasoconstrictors/dilators).
- Optimize cardiac function (e.g. thrombolytic therapy, inotropes, assist devices).

Septic
- Fluids to restore circulating volume.
- Antibiotics or surgery.
- Support cardiac function (e.g. inotropes).

Hypovolaemic
- Identify and arrest losses (may include surgery).
- Restore circulating volume (crystalloids, colloids or blood).
- Support cardiac function.

Deal with the cause of the shock: e.g. stop the bleeding, drain the abscess, remove the source of the anaphylactic antigen, etc.

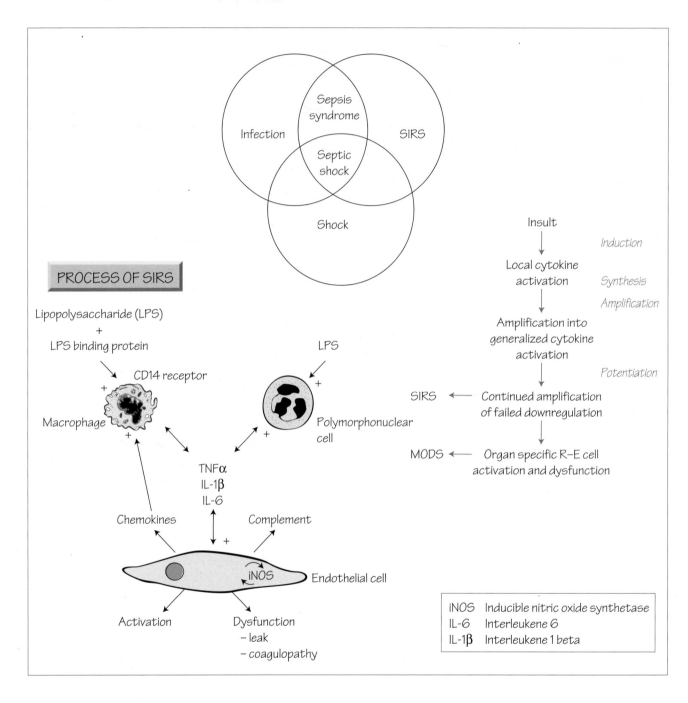

Definitions

SIRS (*systemic inflammatory response syndrome*) is a systemic inflammatory response characterized by the presence of two or more of the following:

- hyperthermia > 38°C or hypothermia < 36°C
- tachycardia > 90 bpm
- tachypnoea > 20 r.p.m. or Pa_{CO_2} < 4.3 kPa
- neutrophilia > 12×10^{-9} l^{-1} or neutropenia < 4×10^{-9} l^{-1}.

Sepsis syndrome is a state of SIRS with proven infection. *Septic shock* is *sepsis* with systemic shock.

MODS (*multiple organ dysfunction syndrome*) is a state of derangement of physiology such that organ function cannot maintain homoeostasis.

The common terminal pathways for organ damage and dysfunction are vasodilatation, capillary leak, intravascular coagulation and endothelial cell activation.

Key points

- SIRS is more common in surgical patients than is diagnosed.
- Early treatment of SIRS may reduce the risk of MODS developing.
- The role of treatment is to eliminate any causative factor and support the cardiovascular and respiratory physiology until the patient can recover.
- Overall mortality is 7% for a diagnosis of SIRS, 14% for sepsis syndrome and 40% for established septic shock.

Common surgical causes

- Acute pancreatitis.
- Perforated viscus with peritonitis.
- Fulminant colitis.
- Multiple trauma.
- Massive blood transfusion.
- Aspiration pneumonia.
- Ischaemia reperfusion injury.

Causation and treatments

TNFα

TNFα is both released by and activates macrophages and neutrophils. It is cytotoxic to endothelial cells and parenchymal cells of end organs. There is no clear evidence that anti-TNFα therapy is effective in SIRS.

Lipopolysaccharide (LPS)

Released from Gram −ve bacterial cell walls, activates macrophages via attachment of LPS binding protein and activation of CD14 molecules on the cell surface. There is no proven value for anti-LPS antibody treatment.

Interleukines

IL-6 and IL-1α cause endothelial cell activation and damage. They promote complement and chemokines release. High-dose intravenous steroids have little role in established SIRS (probably because of multiple pathways of activation). Steroids for early SIRS are unproven.

Platelet-activating factor (PAF)

Implicated particularly in acute pancreatitis, no proven role for anti-PAF antibody treatment.

Inducible nitric oxide synthetase (iNOS)

Synthesized by activated endothelial cells, activates endothelial cells and leucocytes, potent negative ionotrope.

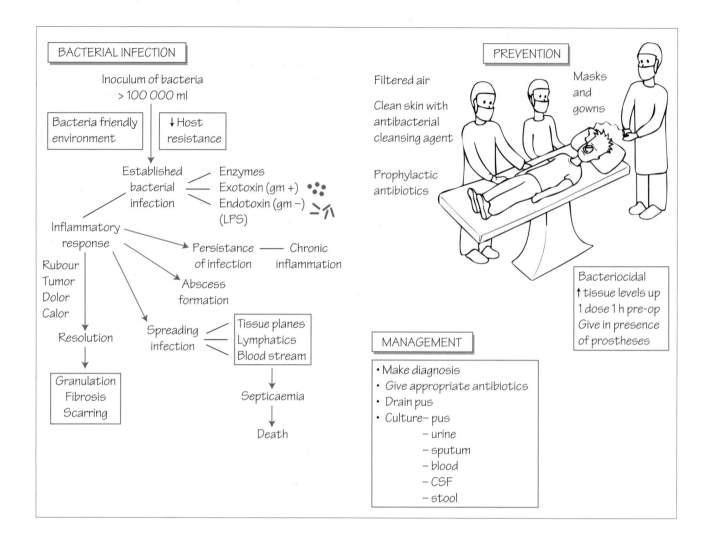

Definitions

Infection is the process whereby organisms (e.g. bacteria, viruses, fungi) capable of causing disease gain access and cause injury or damage to the body or its tissues.

Pus is a yellow/green foul-smelling viscous fluid containing dead leukocytes, bacteria, tissue and protein.

An *abscess* is localized collection of pus, usually surrounded by an intense inflammatory reaction.

Cellulitis is a spreading infection of subcutaneous tissue.

Pathophysiology of bacterial infection

Establishing a bacterial infection requires:
• An inoculum of bacteria, (usually 100 000 organisms per ml of exudate, or gram of tissue, or mm² surface area).
• A bacteria-friendly environment (water, electrolytes, carbohydrate, protein digests, blood).
• Diminished host resistance to infection (impaired physical barriers, reduced biochemical/humoral response, reduced cellular response).

Bacterial secretions

Bacteria cause some of their ill effects by releasing compounds:
• Enzymes (e.g. haemolysin, streptokinase, hyaluronidase).
• Exotoxin (released from intact bacteria, mostly Gram positive, e.g. tetanus, diphtheria.
• Endotoxin (lipopolysaccharides (LPS) released from cell wall on death of bacterium).

Natural history of infection

• Inflammatory response is established: (rubor/redness, tumor/swelling, dolor/pain, calor/heat).
• Resolution: inflammatory reaction settles and infection disappears
• Spreading infection:
  – Direct to adjacent tissues
  – Along tissue planes
  – Via lymphatic system (lymphangitis)
  – Via blood stream
• Abscess formation: Localised collection of pus.
• Organization: Granulation tissue, fibrosis, scarring.

- Chronic infection: persistence of organism in the tissues elicits a chronic inflammatory response.

Koch's postulates for establishing a micro-organism as the cause of a disease
The causative organism:
- is in all patients with the disease
- must be isolated from lesions in pure culture
- must reproduce the disease in susceptible animals
- must be re-isolated from lesions in the experimentally infected animals

---

Management of surgical infection

Preventive measures
- Short operations.
- Skin cleansing with antibacterial chemical and detergents (patient's, surgeons' and nurses' skin).
- Filtering of air in operating theatre.
- Occlusive surgical masks and gowns.
- Prophylactic antibiotics:
  - Should be bacteriocidal.
  - Should have high tissue levels at time of contamination.
  - One pre-operative dose given one hour prior to surgery should suffice unless operation is heavily contaminated or dirty or the patient is immunocompromised.
  - Specific antibiotics should be given to patients with implanted prosthetic materials, e.g. heart valves, vascular grafts, joint prostheses.

Management of established infection
- *Diagnosis* made by culture of appropriate specimens (pus, urine, sputum, blood, CSF, stool).
- *Antibiotics*
  - Prescribe on basis of culture results and 'most likely organism' while waiting for results.
  - Certain antibiotics are reserved for serious infections—use the hospital policy wherever possible.
  - Therapeutic monitoring of drug levels may be required e.g. aminoglycosides.
  - Synergistic combinations may be required in some infections e.g. aminoglycoside, cephalosporin and metronidazole for faecal peritonitis.
  - In serious, atypical or unresponsive infections seek advice from clinical microbiologist.
  - Barrier nursing and isolation of patients with methicillin-resistant *Staphlococcus aureus* (MRSA) or vancomycin resistant enterococcus (VRE).
- *Drainage* surgical or radiological is the most important treatment modality for an abscess or collections of infected fluid.

Wound classification	Definition	Example	Incidence of wound infection %
Clean	No contamination from GI, GU or RT	Thyroidectomy, elective hernia repair	1–5
Clean contaminated	Minimal contamination from GI, GU or RT	Cholecystectomy, TURP, pneumonectomy	7–10
Contaminated	Significantcontamination from GI, GU or RT	Elective colon surgery, inflamed appendicitis	15–20
Dirty	Infection present	Bowel perforation, perforated appendicitis, infected amputation	30–40

Surgical infection—specific

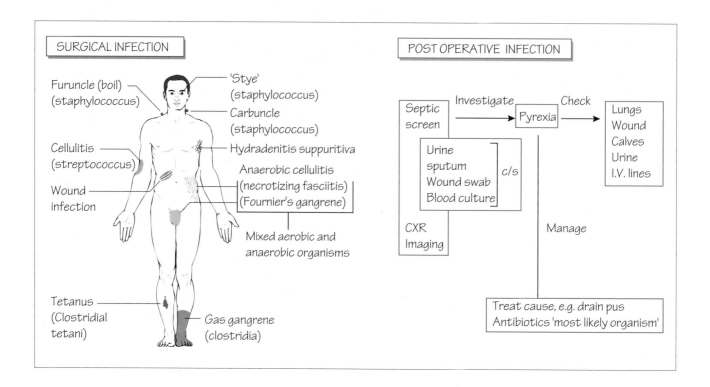

Specific surgical infections
Cellulitis

• Acute pyogenic cellulitis (*Streptococcus pyogenes*). Erysipelas (face) is most virulent form.
• Anaerobic cellulitis. Combination of aerobic and anaerobic organisms. Two forms clinically:
  – Progressive bacterial syergistic gangrene (including Fournier's gangrene).
  – Necrotizing fasciitis.
Staphylococcal infections (*Staphlococcus aureus, Staphlococcus epidermis*).
• Furuncle (a boil)—skin abscess involving hair follicle.
• Stye—infection of eyelash follicle.
• Carabuncle—subcutaneous necrosis with network of small abscesses.
• Sycosis barbae—infection of shaving area caused by infected razor.
Hydradenitis suppuritiva—infection of apocrine glands in skin (axilla, groin).

Tetanus
• Clostridial infection caused by *C. tetani*.
• Penetrating dirty wounds.
• Most symptoms caused by exotoxin which is absorbed by motor nerve endings and migrates to anterior horn cells:
  – Spastic contractions and trismus (lockjaw).
  – Spasm of facial muscles (risus sardonicus).
  – Rigidity and extensor convulsions (opisthotonos).

Standard tetanus prophylaxis in the UK	Tetanus toxoid is given during 1st year of life as part of triple vaccine. Booster at 5 years and end of schooling
• Presentation with potentially contaminated wound + previous full immunization	Booster dose of tetanus toxoid given
• Presentation with potentially contaminated wound – previous immunization	Passive immunization with human antitetanus immunoglobin Full course of active immunization commenced

Gas gangrene
• Clostridial infection caused by *C. perfringes* (65%), *C. Novyi* (30%), *C. Septicum* (15%).
• Contamination of necrotic wounds with soil containing *Clostridia*.
• Spreading gangrene of muscles with crepitus from gas formation, toxaemia and shock.
• Rx—resuscitation, complete debridement and excision of ALL infected tissue (may require several operations).

Post operative infections
Pyrexia is a common sign of infection. A mildly raised temperature is normal in the early post operative period indicating response to major surgery. If pyrexia develops:

Note: • Time of onset (1st 24 h usually atelectasis) • Degree and type: (low persistent = low grade infectivity or inflammatory process, Intermittent = abscess ± rigors or haemodynamic change (bacteraemia/septicaemia)	**Check:** • Lungs (atelectasis/pneumonia) • Wound (infection) • Calves (DVT) • Urine (infection) • I.V. or Central lines
Do: • Septic screen – Urine specimen – Sputum sample – Swabs of wounds or cannulae – Blood cultures • Chest X-ray (± other imaging as indicated e.g. abdominal US or CT scan if peritonitis present)	**Give:** Antibiotics on basis of 'most likely organism' (Refine treatment when septic screen results available) **Treat:** Cause as appropriate (e.g. remove infected cannula, drain abscess surgically or radiologically, give chest physiotherapy respiratory support, deal with anastomotic dehiscence, etc.)

Wound infections
• Incidence depends on wound classification (see above).
• Mild may settle with antibiotics but most need wound to be opened and drained.

Intra-abdominal infections
• Generalized peritonitis—pain, rigidity, absence of bowel sounds.
• Depends on cause—typically: *E Coli*, *Klebsiella*, *Proteus*, *Strep. faecalis*, *Bacteroides*
• Rx—Resuscitation, broad-spectrum antibiotics, laparotomy and deal with cause if appropriate.

Intra-abdominal abscess
• Intermittent pyrexia, localized tenderness ± evidence of bacteraemia/septicaemia.
• Diagnosis by US or CT scanning.
• Rx—Resuscitation, broad-spectrum antibiotics, drainage: either radiologically-guided or open surgical.

Respiratory infections
• Predisposing factors
 – pre-existing pulmonary disease
 – smoking
 – starvation and fluid restriction
 – anaesthesia
 – post operative pain
• Prevention
 – Pre-operative physiotherapy
 – Incentive spirometry
 – Stop smoking
• Treatment

• Physiotherapy and appropriate antibiotics
• Good post-operative analgesia
• Keep well hydrated

Urinary tract infections
• Often related to urinary catheter.
• Only catheterize when necessary.
• Use sterile technique and closed drainage.
• Treat with antibiotic on basis of urine culture.

Intravenous central line infection
• Prevention:
 – Use sterile technique when inserting line.
 – Don't use line for giving i.v. drugs or taking blood samples especially if used for parenteral nutrition.
 – Use single bag parenteral nutrition given over 24 hours.
 – Never add anything to the parenteral nutrition bag.
• Diagnosis:
 – Suspect it with any fever in a patient with a central line.
• Treatment:
 – Remove the line if possible, send tip of catheter for culture, antibiotics (via the line if kept).

Pseudomembranous enterocolitis
• Caused by *Clostridium difficile*.
• Seen in patients who have been on antibiotics (esp cephalosporins).
• Presents with diarrhoea, abdominal discomfort, leukocytosis.
• Dx: clinically—C diff +ve with above clinical picture, pseudomembranous membrane in the colon at endoscopy.
• Rx: resuscitate, stop current antibiotics, oral vancomycin or metronidazole, very rarely life-saving colectomy.

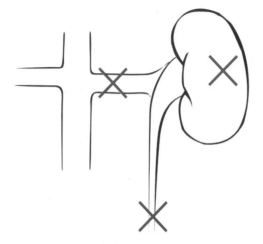

CAUSES

PRE-RENAL
Hypoperfusion
• Hypovolaemia
• Septicaemia
• Hypoxaemia
• Nephrotoxins
• Pancreatitis
• Liver cell dysfunction
    • Bilirubin
    • Other toxins

RENAL
• Any established cause
  of pre-renal or post-renal
• Glomerular damage
    • Glomerulonephritis
• Tubular damage
    • Toxins
    • Drugs
    • Pyelonephritis
• Vascular damage
    • Acute vasculitis
    • Diabetes
    • Hypertension

POST-RENAL
• Primary tumours
• Secondary tumours — invasion
• Stones
• Blood clots
• Bladder obstruction
• Infestations (worms)

FEATURES

	Normal	Prerenal	Renal	Postrenal
$U_{osmolality}$	Approx 400–500 mosm/kg	> 500	< 400	Normal
U_{Na^+}	10–20 mmol/l	< 10	> 20	Normal
U_{urea}/P_{urea}	Approx 5/1	> 10/1	3/1–1/1	Normal
U_{osm}/P_{osm}	Approx 1.5/1	> 2/1	< 1.1/1	Normal
Findings	—	Concentrated urine ? Findings due to cause	Casts RBCs Protein	Normal urine ? Findings due to cause

Definitions

Acute renal failure is a sudden deterioration in renal function such that neither kidney is capable of excreting body waste products (e.g. urea, creatinine, potassium) that accumulate in the blood. It is fatal unless treated. *Anuria* means no urine is passed. *Oliguria* means that less than 0.5 ml/kg/h is passed.

Key points

- Oliguria in a surgical patient is an emergency and the cause must be identified and treated promptly.
- Prompt correction of pre-renal causes may prevent the development of established renal failure.
- Ensure the oliguric patient is normovolaemic as far as possible before starting diuretics or other therapies.
- Don't use blind, large fluid challenges, especially in the elderly—if necessary use a CVP line.
- Established renal failure requires specialist support as electrolyte and fluid imbalances can be rapid in onset and difficult to manage.

Common causes

Pre-renal failure

- Shock causing reduced renal perfusion.
- Pancreatitis.

Intrinsic renal failure

- Shock causing renal ischaemia (ATN).
- Nephrotoxins (aminoglycosides, myoglobin).
- Acute glomerulonephritis.
- Severe pyelonephritis.
- Hypertension and diabetes mellitus.

Post-renal failure

- Urinary tract obstruction, e.g. prostatic hypertrophy.
- Obstructing renal calculi.

Clinical features

Specific to the cause

Hypovolaemia: cool peripheries, tachycardia, confusion, restlessness, dry mucous membranes.

Oliguric phase

(May last hours/days/weeks)
- Oliguria.
- Uraemia: dyspnoea, confusion, drowsiness, coma.
- Nausea, vomiting, hiccoughs, diarrhoea.
- Anaemia, coagulopathy, GI haemorrhage.

- Fluid retention: hypervolaemia, hypertension.
- Hyperkalaemia: dysrrhythmias.
- Acidosis.

Polyuric (recovery) phase

(May last days/weeks)
- Polyuria: hypovolaemia, hypotension.
- Hyponatraemia.
- Hypokalaemia.

Investigations

- Urinalysis (see opposite page).
- U+E (especially K^+).
- Creatinine estimation.
- ECG/chest X-ray.
- Arterial blood gases: metabolic acidosis (N Po_2, Lo Pco_2, Lo pH, Hi base deficit).

Essential management

Prevention

- Keep at-risk patients (e.g. patients with obstructive jaundice) well hydrated pre- and perioperatively.
- Protect renal function in selected patients with drugs such as dopamine and mannitol.
- Monitor renal function regularly in patients on nephrotoxic drugs (e.g. gentamicin).

Identification

- Exclude urinary retention as a cause of anuria by catheterization.
- Correct hypovolaemia as far as possible. Use appropriate fluid boluses—if necessary guided by a CVP monitor.
- A trial of bolus high-dose loop diuretics may be appropriate in a normovolaemic patient.
- Dopamine infusions may be necessary but suggest the need for HDU or ICU care.

Treatment of established renal failure

- Maintain fluid and electrolyte balance.
- Water intake 400 ml/day + measured losses.
- Na^+ intake limited to replace loss only.
- K^+ intake nil (dextrose and insulin and/or ion-exchange resins are required to control hyperkalaemia).
- Diet: high calorie, low protein in a small volume of fluid.
- Acidosis: sodium bicarbonate.
- Treat any infection.
- Dialysis: peritoneal, ultrafiltration, haemodialysis (usually indicated for hypervolaemia, hyperkalaemia or acidosis).

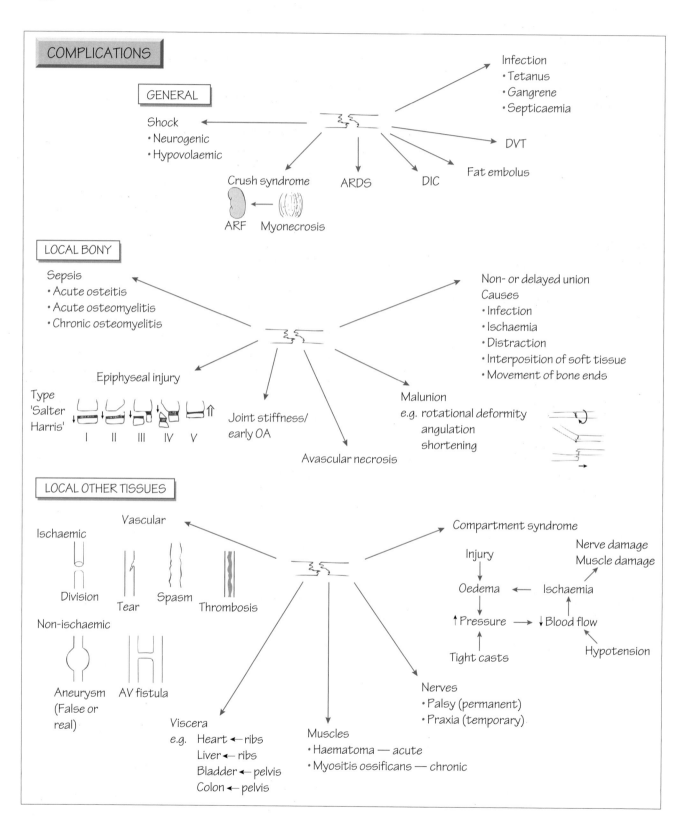

COMPLICATIONS

GENERAL

Infection
• Tetanus
• Gangrene
• Septicaemia

Shock
• Neurogenic
• Hypovolaemic

DVT

Fat embolus

Crush syndrome
ARF ← Myonecrosis

ARDS

DIC

LOCAL BONY

Sepsis
• Acute osteitis
• Acute osteomyelitis
• Chronic osteomyelitis

Non- or delayed union
Causes
• Infection
• Ischaemia
• Distraction
• Interposition of soft tissue
• Movement of bone ends

Epiphyseal injury

Type
'Salter
Harris'   I   II   III   IV   V

Joint stiffness/
early OA

Malunion
e.g. rotational deformity
angulation
shortening

Avascular necrosis

LOCAL OTHER TISSUES

Vascular

Ischaemic

Division   Tear   Spasm   Thrombosis

Non-ischaemic

Aneurysm   AV fistula
(False or
real)

Viscera
e.g. Heart ← ribs
Liver ← ribs
Bladder ← pelvis
Colon ← pelvis

Muscles
• Haematoma — acute
• Myositis ossificans — chronic

Compartment syndrome

Nerve damage
Muscle damage

Injury
↓
Oedema ← Ischaemia
↑
↑Pressure → ↓Blood flow
↑
Tight casts   Hypotension

Nerves
• Palsy (permanent)
• Praxia (temporary)

Definitions

- A *fracture* is a break in the continuity of a bone.
- Fractures may be *transverse*, *oblique* or *spiral* in shape.
- In a *greenstick* fracture, only one side of the bone is fractured, the other simply bends (usually immature bones).
- A *comminuted* fracture is one in which there are more than two fragments of bone.
- In a *complicated* fracture, some other structure is also damaged (e.g. a nerve or blood vessel).
- In a *compound* fracture, there is a break in the overlying skin (or nearby viscera) with potential contamination of the bone ends.
- A *pathological* fracture is one through a bone weakened by disease, e.g. a metastasis.

Key points

- Always consider multiple injury in patients presenting with fractures.
- Compound fractures are a surgical emergency and require appropriate measures to prevent infection, including tetanus prevention.
- Always image the joints above and below a long bone fracture.

Common causes

Fractures occur when excessive force is applied to a normal bone or moderate force to a diseased bone, e.g. osteoporosis.

Clinical features

- Pain.
- Loss of function.
- Deformity, tenderness and swelling.
- Discoloration or bruising.
- (Crepitus, not to be elicited!)

Investigations

- Radiographs in two planes (look for lucencies and discontinuity in the cortex of the bone).
- Tomography, CT scan, MRI scan (rarely).
- Ultrasonography and radioisotope bone scanning. (Bone scan is particularly useful when radiographs/CT scanning are negative in clinically suspect fracture.)

Essential management

General

- Look for shock/haemorrhage and check ABC (see p. 89).
- Look for injury in other areas at risk (head and spine, ribs and pneumothorax, femoral and pelvic injury).

The fracture
Immediate

- Relieve pain (opiates i.v., nerve blocks, splints, traction).
- Establish good i.v. access and send blood for group and crossmatch.
- Open (compound) fractures require débridement, antibiotics and tetanus prophylaxis.

Definitive

- Reduction (closed or open).
- Immobilization (casting, functional bracing, internal fixation, external fixation, traction).
- Rehabilitation (aim to restore the patient to pre-injury level of function with physiotherapy and occupational therapy).

Complications
Early

- Blood loss.
- Infection.
- Fat embolism.
- DVT and PE.
- Renal failure.
- Compartment syndrome.

Late

- Non-union.
- Delayed union.
- Malunion.
- Growth arrest.
- Arthritis.
- Post-traumatic sympathetic (reflex) dystrophy.

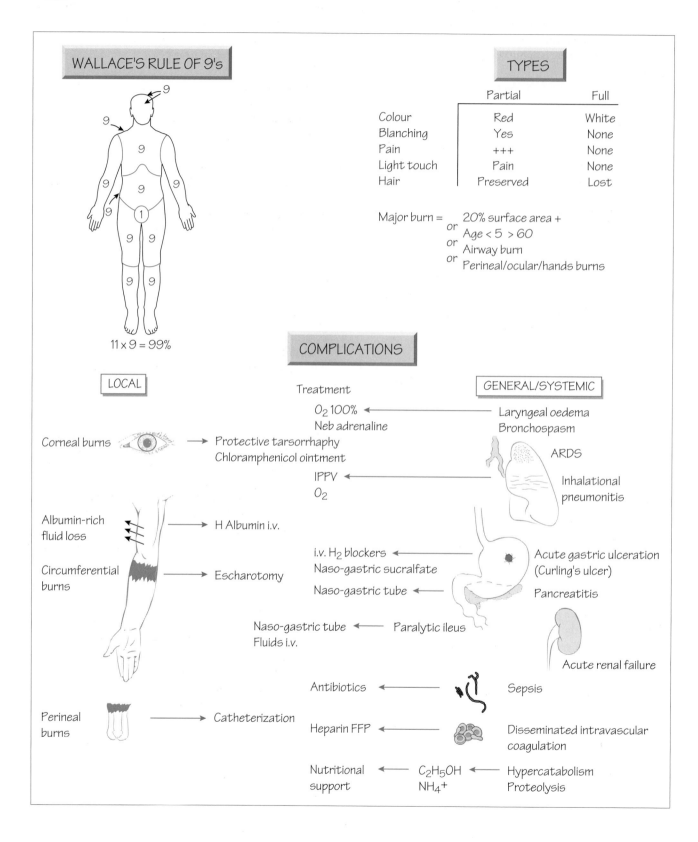

WALLACE'S RULE OF 9's

9
9
9
9 9 9
9 1
9 9
9 9

11 x 9 = 99%

TYPES

	Partial	Full
Colour	Red	White
Blanching	Yes	None
Pain	+++	None
Light touch	Pain	None
Hair	Preserved	Lost

Major burn = or 20% surface area +
or Age < 5 > 60
or Airway burn
or Perineal/ocular/hands burns

COMPLICATIONS

LOCAL

Corneal burns → Protective tarsorrhaphy
Chloramphenicol ointment

Albumin-rich fluid loss → H Albumin i.v.

Circumferential burns → Escharotomy

Perineal burns → Catheterization

Treatment

O_2 100%
Neb adrenaline

IPPV
O_2

i.v. H_2 blockers
Naso-gastric sucralfate

Naso-gastric tube

Naso-gastric tube
Fluids i.v. ← Paralytic ileus

Antibiotics

Heparin FFP

Nutritional support ← C_2H_5OH ←
NH_4^+

GENERAL/SYSTEMIC

Laryngeal oedema
Bronchospasm

ARDS

Inhalational pneumonitis

Acute gastric ulceration (Curling's ulcer)

Pancreatitis

Acute renal failure

Sepsis

Disseminated intravascular coagulation

Hypercatabolism
Proteolysis

Definitions

A *burn* is the response of the skin and subcutaneous tissues to thermal injury. A *partial thickness* burn is a burn that either does not destroy the skin epithelium or destroys only part of it. They usually heal with conservative management. A *full thickness* burn destroys all sources of skin epithelial regrowth and may require excision and skin grafting if large.

Key points

- Start resuscitation immediately in major burns.
- Calculate fluid requirement from the time of the burn.
- Be sure to assess for vital area burns (airway/hands/face/perineum/circumferential).
- Consider referral to a specialist burns centre for all major burns.

Common causes

- Thermal injury from dry (flame, hot metal) or moist (hot liquids or gases) heat sources.
- Electricity (deep burns at entry and exit sites, may cause cardiac arrest).
- Chemicals (usually industrial accidents with acid or alkali).
- Radiation (partial thickness initially, but may progress to chronic deeper injury).

Clinical features

General

- Pain.
- Swelling and blistering.

Specific

- Evidence of smoke inhalation (soot in nose or sputum, burns in the mouth, hoarseness).
- Eye or eyelid burns (early ophthalmological opinion).
- Circumferential burns (will need escharotomy).

Investigations

- FBC.
- U+E.
- If inhalation suspected: chest X-ray, arterial blood gases, CO estimation.
- Blood group and crossmatch.
- ECG/cardiac enzymes with electrical burns.

Complications

Immediate

Compartment syndrome from circumferential burns (limb burns → limb ischaemia, thoracic burns → hypoxia from restrictive respiratory failure) (prevent by urgent escharotomy).

Early

- Hyperkalaemia (from cytolysis in large burns). Treat with insulin and dextrose.
- Acute renal failure (combination of hypovolaemia, sepsis, tissue toxins). Prevent by aggressive early resuscitation, ensuring high GFR with fluid loading and diuretics, treat sepsis.
- Infection (beware of *Streptococcus*). Treat established infection (10^6 organisms present in wound biopsy) with systemic antibiotics.
- Stress ulceration (Curling's ulcer) (prevent with antacid, H_2-blocker or proton pump inhibitor prophylaxis).

Late

Contractures.

Essential management

General

- Start resuscitation (ABC (see p. 89), set up good i.v. lines, give O_2).
- Assess size of burn (Wallace's rule of 9s).

Major burns (> 20% burn in adult, > 10% in child)

- Monitor pulse, BP, temperature, urinary output, give adequate analgesia i.v., consider nasogastric tube, give tetanus prophylaxis.
- Give i.v. fluids according to Muir–Barclay formula:
  % burn × wt in kg/2 = one aliquot of fluid.
  Give six aliquots of fluid over first 36 h in 4, 4, 4, 6, 6, 12-hour sequence from time of burn. Colloid, albumin or plasma solutions are used.
- The burn wound is treated as for minor burns (see below).
- Consider referral to a burns centre.

Minor burns (< 20% burn in adult, < 10% in child)

- Treatment by exposure—débride wound and leave exposed in special clean environment.
- Treatment by dressings—cover with tulle gras impregnated with chlorhexidine or silver sulphadiazine under absorptive gauze dressings.
- Débridement of eschar and split skin grafting.

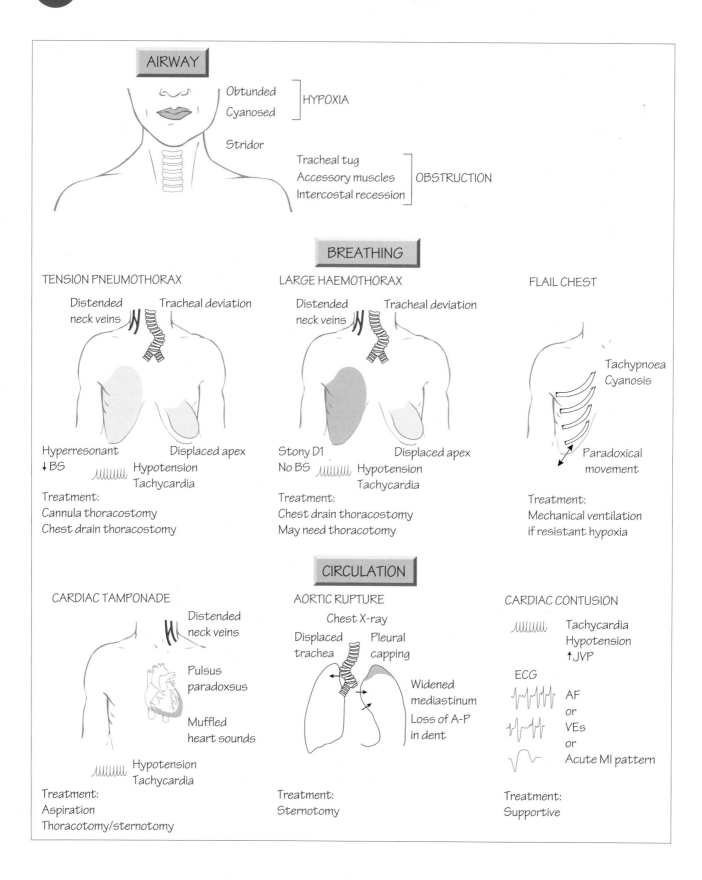

AIRWAY

Obtunded
Cyanosed] HYPOXIA

Stridor

Tracheal tug
Accessory muscles] OBSTRUCTION
Intercostal recession

BREATHING

TENSION PNEUMOTHORAX

Distended neck veins   Tracheal deviation

Hyperresonant   Displaced apex
↓BS   Hypotension
          Tachycardia

Treatment:
Cannula thoracostomy
Chest drain thoracostomy

LARGE HAEMOTHORAX

Distended neck veins   Tracheal deviation

Stony D1   Displaced apex
No BS   Hypotension
          Tachycardia

Treatment:
Chest drain thoracostomy
May need thoracotomy

FLAIL CHEST

Tachypnoea
Cyanosis

Paradoxical movement

Treatment:
Mechanical ventilation
if resistant hypoxia

CIRCULATION

CARDIAC TAMPONADE

Distended neck veins

Pulsus paradoxsus

Muffled heart sounds

Hypotension
Tachycardia

Treatment:
Aspiration
Thoracotomy/sternotomy

AORTIC RUPTURE

Chest X-ray
Displaced   Pleural
trachea   capping

Widened mediastinum
Loss of A-P in dent

Treatment:
Sternotomy

CARDIAC CONTUSION

Tachycardia
Hypotension
↑JVP

ECG

AF
or
VEs
or
Acute MI pattern

Treatment:
Supportive

Definition

Major trauma (MT) can be defined as injury (or injuries) of organs of severity sufficient to present an immediate threat to life. MT often involves multiple injuries. The majority of patients who reach hospital alive following MT have potentially survivable injuries if detected and treated early.

Key points

- Treat all MT patients as having a potentially unstable cervical spine.
- Treat life-threatening injuries identified in the primary survey immediately upon discovery.
- Undiagnosed hypotension is due to occult haemorrhage unless proven otherwise.
- Emergency surgery may be part of the resuscitation of patients suffering from internal haemorrhage.

Principles of management

Management for MT is divided into two categories.
- **'First aid'**—'roadside' given by paramedics or on-site medical teams. Aims to maintain life during extraction and evacuation of patient.
- **Primary survey**—in hospital performed by A&E or Trauma Teams. Aims to identify and treat life-threatening injuries to airways, respiratory and cardiovascular systems and perform major skeletal radiology. Known as the ABC(DE) **secondary survey**—in hospital performed by A&E or Trauma Teams, possibly with specialist surgical staff. Aims to identify and assess all major injuries.

Patterns of injury

Some of the major injuries which may be encountered in the primary survey are shown opposite. Mechanisms of injury and patterns of injury may be associated, e.g.

Restrained RTA	Pedestrian collision
Cervical spine injury	Long bone fractures
Sternal fracture	Knee ligamentous injury
Cardiac contusion	Rib fractures
Liver laceration	Pneumothorax
	Facial fractures
	Head injury

Essential primary survey management

Cervical spine

- Stabilize with in-line manual traction.	Lateral C spine/X-ray (must include C7–T1)
- Secure with hard collar, head supports and tape.	
- Can only be 'cleared' by normal examination in a fully conscious patient or normal X-rays.	

A Airway management (see opposite for major abnormalities)
- Clear obstructions by hand and lift chin (obtunded patients).
- Secure airway with oropharyngeal or nasopharyngeal airway (obtunded patients).
- Definitive airway (direct access to intratracheal oxygenation) indicated by:
  Apnoea / (risk of) upper airway obstruction / (risk of) aspiration / need for mechanical ventilation.
  Orotracheal tube.
  Nasotracheal tube.
- Surgical airway (cricothyroidotomy) indicated by:
  Maxillofacial injuries/laryngeal disruption/failure to intubate.

B Breathing (see opposite for some major abnormalities)

- Administer supplemental O_2.	
- Assess respiratory rate / air entry (symmetry)/chest wall motion (symmetry)/tracheal position.	CXR
- Monitor with pulse oximetry and observations.	

C Circulation (see opposite for some major abnormalities)

- Assess pulse rate and character/blood pressure/apex beat/JVP/heart sounds/evidence of blood loss.	Pelvic X-ray
- Draw blood for cross match, FBC and U+E.	

D Dysfunction of the CNS
- Assess GCS (see p. 81)/pupil reactivity/limb gross motor and sensory function where possible.

E Exposure of extremities
- Assess limbs for major long bone injuries and sites of major blood loss.

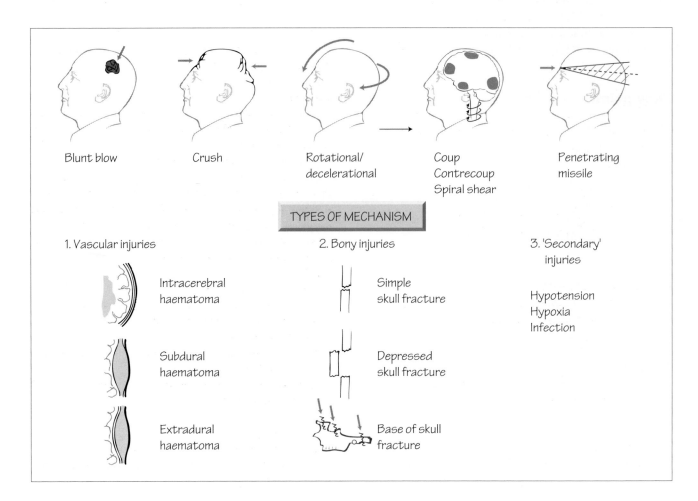

Blunt blow

Crush

Rotational/
decelerational

Coup
Contrecoup
Spiral shear

Penetrating
missile

TYPES OF MECHANISM

1. Vascular injuries

Intracerebral
haematoma

Subdural
haematoma

Extradural
haematoma

2. Bony injuries

Simple
skull fracture

Depressed
skull fracture

Base of skull
fracture

3. 'Secondary'
injuries

Hypotension
Hypoxia
Infection

Definitions

• A *head injury* is the process whereby direct or decelerating trauma to the head results in skull and brain damage.
• *Primary brain injury* is the damage that occurs to the brain immediately as the result of the trauma.
• *Secondary brain injury* is the damage that develops later as a result of complications.

Key points

• Prevention of secondary brain injury is the most important objective of head injury care.
• A full trauma survey (p. 89) must be carried out on all patients with head injuries.
• The Glasgow Coma Scale (GCS) provides a simple method of monitoring global CNS function over a period rather than a precise index of brain injury at any one time.

Epidemiology

Head injury is very common. A million patients each year present to A&E departments in the UK with head injury and about 5000 patients die each year following head injuries.

Pathophysiology

Direct blow

May cause damage to the brain at the site of the blow (*coup injury*) or to the side opposite the blow when the brain moves within the skull and hits the opposite wall (*contrecoup injury*).

Rotation/deceleration

Neck flexion, extension or rotation results in the brain striking bony points within the skull (e.g. the wing of the sphenoid bone).

Severe rotation also causes shear injuries within the white matter of the brain and brainstem, causing axonal injury and intracerebral petechial haemorrhages.

Crush

The brain is often remarkably spared direct injury unless severe (especially in children with elastic skulls).

Missiles

Tend to cause loss of tissue with injury proportionate. Brain swelling less of a problem due to the skull disruption automatically decompressing the brain!
• The degree of primary brain injury is directly related to the amount of force applied to the head.
• Secondary damage results from: respiratory complications (*hypoxia, hypercarbia, airway obstruction*), hypovolaemic shock (head injury does not cause hypovolaemic shock—look for another cause), intracranial bleeding, cerebral oedema, epilepsy, infection and hydrocephalus.

Clinical features

• History of direct trauma to head or deceleration.
• Patient must be assessed fully for other injuries.
• Level of consciousness determined by GCS.
• Pupillary inequalities or abnormal light reflex indicate intracranial haemorrhage.
• Headache, nausea, vomiting, a falling pulse rate and rising BP indicate cerebral oedema.

Investigations

• Skull X-ray: AP, lateral and Towne's views.
• CT/MRI scan: show contusions, haematomas, hydrocephalus, cerebral oedema.

The Glasgow Coma Scale.

Eye opening	Voice response	Best motor response
Spontaneous 4	Alert and orientated 5	Obeys commands 6
To voice 3	Confused 4	Localizes pain 5
To pain 2	Inappropriate 3	Flexes to pain 4
No eye opening 1	Incomprehensible 2	Abnormal flexion to pain 3
	No voice response 1	Extends to pain 2
		No response to pain 1

Fully conscious: GCS = 15; deep coma: GCS = 3.

Head injury/2

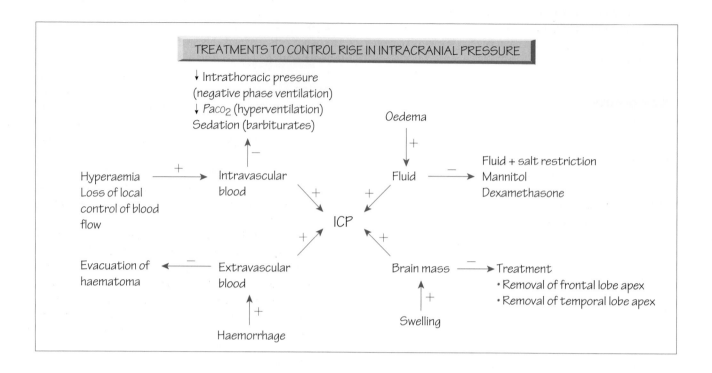

TREATMENTS TO CONTROL RISE IN INTRACRANIAL PRESSURE

↓ Intrathoracic pressure
(negative phase ventilation)
↓ Pa_{CO_2} (hyperventilation)
Sedation (barbiturates)

Oedema

Hyperaemia
Loss of local
control of blood
flow
— + → Intravascular
blood

Fluid — − → Fluid + salt restriction
Mannitol
Dexamethasone

ICP

Evacuation of ← − Extravascular
haematoma   blood

Brain mass — − → Treatment
• Removal of frontal lobe apex
• Removal of temporal lobe apex

Swelling

Haemorrhage

Essential management

Trivial head injury

The patient is conscious, may be history of period of loss of consciousness (LOC). Retrograde amnesia for events prior to head injury is significant.

Indications for skull X-ray

- LOC or amnesia.
- Neurological signs.
- CSF leakage.
- Suspected penetrating injury.
- Alcohol intoxication.
- Difficulty in assessing patient.

Indications for admission

- Confusion or reduced GCS.
- Skull fracture.
- Neurological signs or headache or vomiting.
- Difficulty in assessing patient.
- Coexisting medical problem.
- Inadequate social conditions or lack of responsible adult to observe patient.

Indications for neurosurgical referral

- Skull fracture + confusion/decreasing GCS.
- Focal neurological signs or fits.
- Persistence of neurological signs or confusion for >12 h.
- Coma after resuscitation.
- Suspected open injury to skull.
- Depressed skull fracture.
- Deterioration.

Severe head injury

- Patient will arrive unconscious in A&E department. Head injury may be part of a multiple trauma.
- ABC (see p. 89). Intubate and ventilate unconscious patients to protect airway and prevent secondary brain injury from hypoxia.
- Resuscitate patient and look for other injuries, especially if the patient is in shock. Head injury may be accompanied by cervical spine injury and the neck must be protected by a cervical collar in these patients.
- Treat life-threatening problems (e.g. ruptured spleen) and stabilize patient before transfer to neurosurgical unit. Ensure adequate medical supervision (anaesthetist + nurse) during transfer.

Complications
Skull fractures

Indicate severity of injury. No specific treatment required unless compound, depressed or associated with chronic CSF loss (e.g. anterior cranial fossa basal skull fracture).

Intracranial haemorrhage

- Extradural haemorrhage: tear in middle meningeal artery. Haematoma between skull and dura. Often a 'lucid interval' before signs of raised intracranial pressure (ICP) ensue (falling pulse, rising BP, ipsilateral pupillary dilatation, contralateral paresis or paralysis). Treatment is by evacuation of haematoma via burr holes.
- Acute subdural haemorrhage: tearing of veins between arachnoid and dura mater. Usually seen in elderly. Progressive neurological deterioration. Treatment is by evacuation but even then recovery may be incomplete.
- Chronic subdural haematoma: tear in vein leads to subdural haematoma which enlarges slowly by absorption of CSF. Often the precipitating injury is trivial. Drowsiness and confusion, headache, hemiplegia. Treatment is by evacuation of the clot.
- Intracerebral haemorrhage: haemorrhage into brain substance causes irreversible damage. Efforts are made to avoid secondary injury by ensuring adequate oxygenation and nutrition.

Prognosis

Prognosis is related to level of consciousness on arrival in hospital.

GCS on admission	Mortality
15	1%
8–12	5%
<8	40%

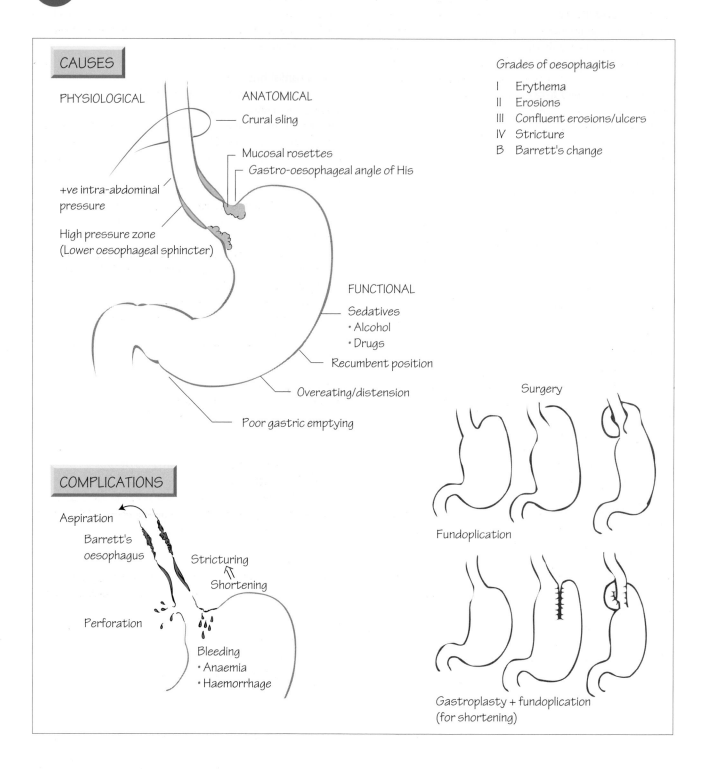

CAUSES

PHYSIOLOGICAL

ANATOMICAL

Crural sling

Mucosal rosettes

Gastro-oesophageal angle of His

+ve intra-abdominal pressure

High pressure zone (Lower oesophageal sphincter)

FUNCTIONAL

Sedatives
• Alcohol
• Drugs

Recumbent position

Overeating/distension

Poor gastric emptying

Grades of oesophagitis

I Erythema
II Erosions
III Confluent erosions/ulcers
IV Stricture
B Barrett's change

Surgery

Fundoplication

Gastroplasty + fundoplication (for shortening)

COMPLICATIONS

Aspiration

Barrett's oesophagus

Stricturing

Shortening

Perforation

Bleeding
• Anaemia
• Haemorrhage

Definitions

Gastro-oesophageal reflux is a condition caused by the retrograde passage of gastric contents into the oesophagus resulting in inflammation (*oesophagitis*), which manifests as dyspepsia. A *hiatus hernia* is an abnormal protrusion of the proximal stomach through the oesophageal opening in the diaphragm resulting in a more proximal positioning of the oesophagogastric junction and predisposition to gastro-oesophageal reflux disease (GORD). *Sliding* (common) and *rolling* or *para-oesophageal* (rare) hiatus hernias are recognized.

Key points

- The majority of GORD is benign and uncomplicated.
- Barrett's oesophagus is an increasingly recognized association predisposing to adenocarcinoma of the oesophagus.
- Patients over the 45 years or with suspicious symptoms should have malignancy excluded as a cause when first presenting with GORD symptoms.
- Surgery for GORD should be reserved for complications or patients resistant to medical therapy.

Common causes

- Failure of normal mechanisms of gastro-oesophageal continence (LOS pressure, length of intra-abdominal LOS, angle of His, sling fibres around the cardia, the crural fibres of the diaphragm, the mucosal rosette).
- LOS pressure reduced by smoking, alcohol and coffee.

Clinical features

- Retrosternal burning pain, radiating to epigastrium, jaw and arms. (Oesophageal pain is often confused with cardiac pain.)
- Regurgitation of acid contents into the mouth (waterbrash).
- Back pain (a penetrating ulcer in Barrett's oesophagus).
- Dysphagia from a benign stricture.

Investigations

- Barium swallow and meal: sliding hiatus hernia, oesophageal ulcer, stricture.
- Oesophagoscopy: assess oesophagitis, biopsy for histology, dilate stricture if present.
- 24-hour pH monitoring: assess the degree of reflux.
- Oesophageal manometry.

Essential management

General

- Lose weight, avoid smoking, coffee, alcohol and chocolate.
- Avoid tight garments and stooping.

Medical

- Exclude carcinoma by OGD in patients over 45 years and with symptoms suspicious of malignancy.
- Control acid secretion (H_2 receptor antagonists (e.g. ranitidine) or proton pump inhibitors (PPIs) (e.g. omeprazole)).
- Minimize effects of reflux (give alginates to protect oesophagus).
- Prokinetic agents (e.g. metoclopramide, cisapride) improve LOS tone and promote gastric emptying.

Surgical

- Anti reflux surgery (e.g. Nissen fundoplication) which may be performed by laparotomy or laparoscopy. Indicated for:
    complications of reflux;
    failed medical control of symptoms;
    ?long-term dependence on medical treatment;
    ?'large volume' reflux.

Complications

- Benign stricture of the oesophagus.
- Barrett's oesophagus (see below).
- Bleeding.

Barrett's oesophagus

Definition and aetiology

>3 cm of columnar epithelium lining the lower anatomical oesophagus. May be related to eradication of *Helicobacter pylori* and increasing incidence of GORD.

Diagnosis

Can only be confidently made by biopsy but appearances of 'reddish' mucosa in the lower oesophagus are typical on OGD.

Complications

Risk of adenocarcinoma:

- 2%—no dysplasia present;
- 20%—low-grade dysplasia present;
- 50%—high-grade dysplasia present.

Treatment

- Follow-up OGD (close surveillance if low-grade dysplasia) and PPI/H_2 blockers.
- Oesophagectomy if high-grade dysplasia due to risk of carcinoma.

40 Oesophageal carcinoma

TYPES

Malignant stricture

Malignant ulcer

Invasive mass

EFFECTS/SPREAD

Supraclavicular node (Virchow's)

Dyspnoea
Cough
Haemoptysis

Mediastinal nodes

AF
Pericardial effusion

Pleural effusion

Gastric nodes

Dysphagia
Dyspepsia

DISTRIBUTION

Postcricoid (10%) – Squamous carcinoma
• Iron deficiency
• Smoking

Upper/middle 1/3 (40%) – Squamous carcinoma
• Smoking
• Diet
• Achalasia

Lower 1/3 (50%) – Squamous/adeno carcinoma
• Barrett's oesophagus

SURGICAL OPTIONS

Lower 1/3 OGJ
(large stomach element)

Total gastrectomy
+ Roux-en-y loop

Lower/middle 1/3

Oesophago-
gastrectomy

Upper 1/3

Oesophagectomy +
interposition graft

Postcricoid

Pharyngo(laryngo)
oesophagectomy +
interposition graft

Definition

Malignant lesion of the epithelial lining of the oesophagus.

Key points

- All new symptoms of dysphagia should raise the possibility of oesophageal carcinoma.
- Adenocarcinoma of the oesophagus is increasingly common.
- Only a minority of tumours are successfully cured by surgery.

Epidemiology

- Male/female 3 : 1, peak incidence 50–70 years. High incidence in areas of China, Russia, Scandinavia and among the Bantu in South Africa.
- Adenocarcinoma has the fastest increasing incidence of any carcinoma in the UK.

Aetiology

The following are predisposing factors.
- Alcohol consumption and cigarette smoking.
- Chronic oesophagitis and Barrett's oesophagus.
- Stricture from corrosive (lye) oesophagitis.
- Achalasia.
- Plummer–Vinson syndrome (oesophageal web, mucosal lesions of mouth and pharynx, iron deficiency anaemia).
- Nitrosamines.

Pathology

- Histological type: 90% squamous carcinoma (upper two-thirds of oesophagus); 10% adenocarcinoma (lower third of oesophagus).
- Spread: lymphatics, direct extension, vascular invasion.

Clinical features

- Dysphagia progressing from solids to liquids.
- Weight loss and weakness.
- Aspiration pneumonia.

Investigations

- Barium swallow: narrowed lumen with 'shouldering'.
- Oesophagoscopy and biopsy: malignant stricture. (Transluminal ultrasound may help assess local invasion.)
- Bronchoscopy: assess bronchial invasion with upper third lesions.
- CT scanning (helical): assess degree of spread if surgery is being contemplated.
- Laparoscopy to assess liver and peritoneal involvement prior to proceeding to surgery.

Essential management

Palliation
- Intubation with Atkinson or Celestine tube endoprosthesis (rarely used).
Self expanding metal stents.
- Radiotherapy—external beam DXT or occasionally intraluminal with iridium wires.
- Laser resection of the tumour to create lumen.

Curative treatment
- Surgical resection is potentially curative only if lymph nodes are not involved and clear tumours margins can be achieved. Neoadjuvant treatment is often given in the form of chemoradiotherapy.
- Reconstruction is by jejunal or gastric 'pull-up' or rarely colon interposition.

Prognosis

Following resection, 5-year survival rates are about 15%, but overall 5-year survival (palliation and resection) is only about 4%.

2 Week wait referral criteria for suspected upper GI cancer

- New onset dysphagia (any age)
- Dyspepsia + wieght loss/anaemia/vomitting
- Dyspepsia + FHx/Barrett's oesophagis/previous peptic ulcer surgery/atrophic gastritis/pernicious anaemia
- New dyspepsia > 55 years
- Jaundice
- Upper abdominal mass

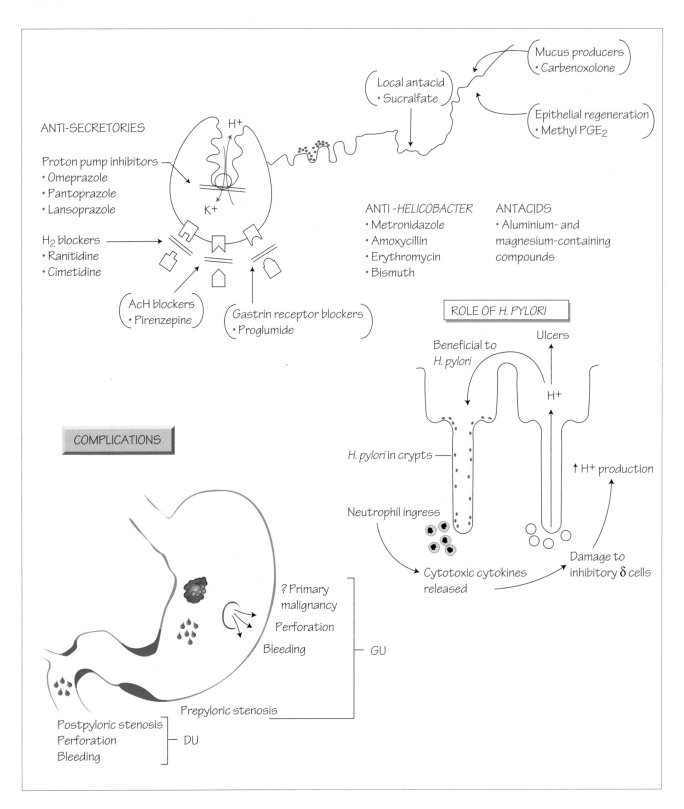

ANTI-SECRETORIES

Proton pump inhibitors
• Omeprazole
• Pantoprazole
• Lansoprazole

H$_2$ blockers
• Ranitidine
• Cimetidine

AcH blockers
• Pirenzepine

Gastrin receptor blockers
• Proglumide

Local antacid
• Sucralfate

Mucus producers
• Carbenoxolone

Epithelial regeneration
• Methyl PGE$_2$

ANTI -HELICOBACTER
• Metronidazole
• Amoxycillin
• Erythromycin
• Bismuth

ANTACIDS
• Aluminium- and magnesium-containing compounds

ROLE OF H. PYLORI

Beneficial to H. pylori

Ulcers

H. pylori in crypts

H$^+$

Neutrophil ingress

↑ H$^+$ production

Cytotoxic cytokines released

Damage to inhibitory δ cells

COMPLICATIONS

? Primary malignancy
Perforation
Bleeding
— GU

Prepyloric stenosis

Postpyloric stenosis
Perforation
Bleeding
— DU

Definition

A *peptic ulcer* is a break in the epithelial surface of the oesophagus, stomach or duodenum (rarely Meckel's diverticulum) caused by the action of gastric secretions (acid and pepsin) and, in the case of duodenal ulceration, infection with *Helicobacter pylori*.

Key points

- Not all dyspepsia is due to PUD.
- The majority of chronic duodenal ulcers are related to *H. pylori* infection and respond to eradication therapy.
- All patients over 45 years at presentation or with suspicious symptoms require endoscopy to exclude malignancy.
- Surgery is usually limited to complications of ulcer disease and failure of compliant medical therapy.

Common causes

- Imbalance between acid/pepsin secretion and mucosal defence.
- Acid hypersecretion occurs because of increased numbers of parietal cells (or rarely in response to gastrin hypersecretion in the Zollinger–Ellison syndrome).
- Defects in mucosal defence (e.g. mucus secretion).
- NSAIDs and the usual suspects: alcohol, cigarettes and 'stress'!
- Infection with *H. pylori*.

Clinical features

Duodenal ulcer and type II gastric ulcer (i.e. prepyloric and antral)

- Male/female 4 : 1, peak incidence 25–50 years.
- Epigastric pain during fasting (hunger pain), relieved by food/antacids, typically exhibits periodicity.
- Boring back pain if ulcer is penetrating posteriorly.
- Haematemesis from ulcer penetrating gastroduodenal artery posteriorly.
- Peritonitis if perforation occurs with anterior duodenal ulcer.
- Vomiting if gastric outlet obstruction (pyloric stenosis) occurs (note succussion splash and watch for hypokalaemic, hypochloraemic alkalosis).

Type I gastric ulcer (i.e. body of stomach)

- Male/female 3 : 1, peak incidence 50+ years.
- Epigastric pain induced by eating.
- Weight loss.

- Nausea and vomiting.
- Anaemia from chronic blood loss.

Investigations

- FBC: to check for anaemia.
- U+E: rarely indicates Zollinger–Ellison syndrome.
- Faecal occult blood.
- OGD: necessary to exclude malignant gastric ulcer in:
  patients over 45 at first presentation;
  concomitant anaemia;
  short history of symptoms;
  other symptoms suggestive of malignancy.
- Useful to obtain biopsy for *Campylobacter*-like organism (CLO) (urease) test.
- Barium meal: best for patients unable to tolerate OGD or evaluation of the duodenum in cases of pyloric stenosis.
- Urease breath test/*H. pylori* serology: non-invasive method of assessing the presence of *H. pylori* infection. Used to direct therapy or confirm eradication.

Essential management

Medical

- Avoid smoking and foods that cause pain.
- Antacids for symptomatic relief.
- H_2 blockers (ranitidine, cimetidine).
- PPIs (omeprazole).
- Colloidal bismuth.
- Ampicillin or tetracycline + metronidazole.
(These are effective against *Helicobacter pylori*.)
- Re-endoscope patients with gastric ulcer after 6 weeks because of risk of malignancy.

Surgical

- Only indicated for failure of medical treatment and complications.
- Elective for duodenal ulcer: highly selective vagotomy; rarely performed now.
- Elective for gastric ulcer: Billroth I gastrectomy.
- Perforated duodenal/gastric ulcer: simple closure of perforation and biopsy.
- Haemorrhage: endoscopic control by sclerotherapy, undersewing bleeding vessel ± vagotomy.
- Pyloric stenosis: gastroenterostomy ± truncal vagotomy.

TNM STAGING

N_1 (Local, ~3 cm) N_2 (Regional, 3 cm+) N_3 (Distant)

T_1 — Mucosal invasion
T_2 — Into muscularis propria
T_3 — Across muscularis propria
T_4 — Onto serosa/organ invasion

PROGNOSIS

Stage		5-year survival
1	$T_{1-2} N_0 M_0$	75%
2	$T_{1-4} N_{1-2} M_0$	35%
3	$T_{1-3} N_{1-3} M_0$	10%
4	$T_4 N_3 M_1$	2%

TYPES OF TUMOUR

Infiltrating mass
Oesophageal obstruction
Malignant polyp
Pyloric obstruction
Malignant ulcer
Linitus plastica

SITES OF SPREAD

Diaphragm
Retro-peritoneum
Spleen
Pylorus
Pancreas
Transverse colon
Omentum
Peritoneum + ovary

TYPES OF OPERATION

Extent of resection

Total gastrectomy + Roux-en-y oesophagojejunostomy

Bilroth I partial gastrectomy

Polya partial gastrectomy

PALLIATIVE TREATMENT

Gastrojejunostomy

Laser therapy (oesophageal obstruction)
Chemotherapy
Alcohol injection (bleeding)

Definition
Malignant lesion of the stomach epithelium.

Key points

- The majority of tumours are unresectable at presentation.
- Tumours considered candidates for resection should be staged with CT and laparoscopy to reduce the risk of an 'open and shut' laparotomy.
- Most tumours are poorly responsive to chemotherapy.

Epidemiology
Male/female 2 : 1, peak incidence 50+ years. Incidence has decreased in Western world over last 50 years. Still common in Japan, Chile and Scandinavia.

Aetiology
The following are predisposing factors.
- Diet (smoked fish, pickled vegetables, benzpyrene, nitrosamines).
- Atrophic gastritis.
- Pernicious anaemia.
- Previous partial gastrectomy.
- Familial hypogammaglobulinaemia.
- Gastric adenomatous polyps.
- Blood group A.

Pathology
- Histology: adenocarcinoma.
- Advanced gastric cancer (penetrated muscularis propria) may be polypoid, ulcerating or infiltrating (i.e. linitus plastica).
- Early gastric cancer (confined to mucosa or submucosa).
- Spread: lymphatic (e.g. Virchow's node); haematogenous to liver, lung, brain; transcoelomic to ovary (Krukenberg tumour).

Clinical features
- History of recent dyspepsia (epigastric discomfort, postprandial fullness, loss of appetite).
- Anaemia.
- Dysphagia.
- Vomiting.
- Weight loss.
- The presence of physical signs usually indicates advanced (incurable) disease.

Investigations
- FBC.
- U+E.
- LFTs.
- OGD (see the lesion and obtain biopsy to distinguish from benign gastric ulcer).
- Barium meal (space-occupying lesion/ulcer with rolled edge). Best for patients unable to tolerate OGD.
- CT scan (helical): stages disease locally and systemically.
- Laparoscopy: used to exclude undiagnosed peritoneal or liver secondaries prior to consideration of resection.

Essential management

- Palliation (metastatic disease or gross distal nodal disease at presentation):
    gastrectomy: local symptoms, e.g. bleeding;
    gastroenterostomy: malignant pyloric obstruction;
    intubation: obstructing lesions at the cardia.
- Curative treatment (resectable primary and local nodes).
- Surgical excision with clear margins and locoregional lymph node clearance (D2 gastrectomy).
- Other treatment: combination chemotherapy with etoposide, adriamycin and cisplatin may induce regression.

Prognosis
Following 'curative' resection, 5-year survival rates are approximately 20%, but overall 5-year survival (palliation and resection) is only about 5%.

2 Week wait referral criteria for suspected upper GI cancer

- New onset dysphagia (any age)
- Dyspepsia + weight loss/anaemia/vomitting
- Dyspepsia + FHx/Barrett's oesophagus/previous peptic ulcer surgery/atrophic gastritis/pernicious anaemia
- New dyspepsia > 55 years
- Jaundice
- Upper abdominal mass

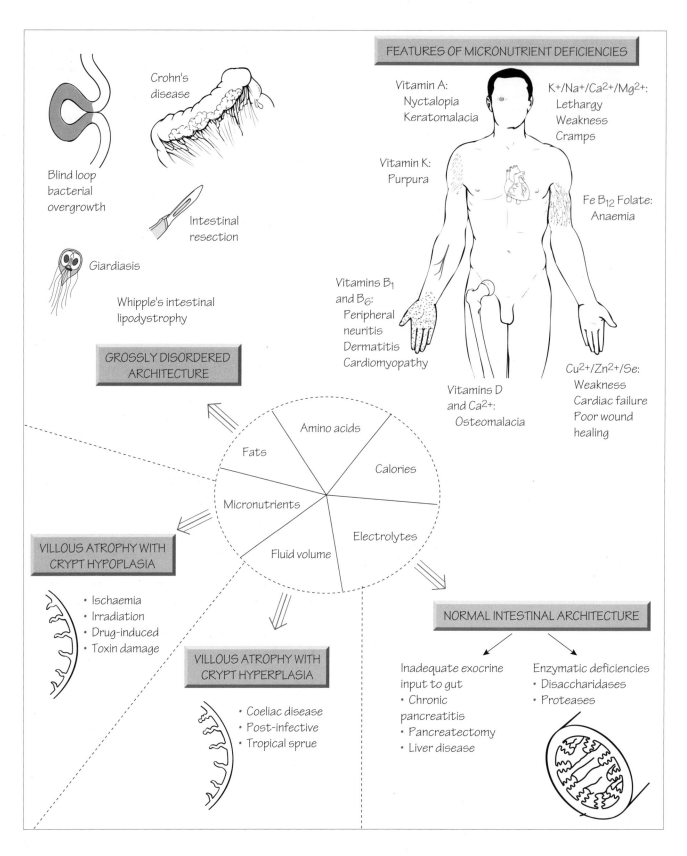

Crohn's disease

Blind loop bacterial overgrowth

Intestinal resection

Giardiasis

Whipple's intestinal lipodystrophy

GROSSLY DISORDERED ARCHITECTURE

FEATURES OF MICRONUTRIENT DEFICIENCIES

Vitamin A:
Nyctalopia
Keratomalacia

$K^+/Na^+/Ca^{2+}/Mg^{2+}$:
Lethargy
Weakness
Cramps

Vitamin K:
Purpura

Fe B_{12} Folate:
Anaemia

Vitamins B_1 and B_6:
Peripheral neuritis
Dermatitis
Cardiomyopathy

Vitamins D and Ca^{2+}:
Osteomalacia

$Cu^{2+}/Zn^{2+}/Se$:
Weakness
Cardiac failure
Poor wound healing

Amino acids

Fats

Calories

Micronutrients

Electrolytes

Fluid volume

VILLOUS ATROPHY WITH CRYPT HYPOPLASIA

• Ischaemia
• Irradiation
• Drug-induced
• Toxin damage

VILLOUS ATROPHY WITH CRYPT HYPERPLASIA

• Coeliac disease
• Post-infective
• Tropical sprue

NORMAL INTESTINAL ARCHITECTURE

Inadequate exocrine input to gut
• Chronic pancreatitis
• Pancreatectomy
• Liver disease

Enzymatic deficiencies
• Disaccharidases
• Proteases

Definition

Malabsorption is the failure of the body to acquire and conserve adequate amounts of one or more essential dietary elements. The cause may be localized or generalized.

Key points

- Malabsorption usually affects several nutrient groups.
- Coeliac disease is a common cause and may present with obscure, vague abdominal symptoms.
- Always consider micronutrients and trace elements in malabsorption.

Differential diagnosis

Coeliac disease

- Classically presents as sensitivity to gluten-containing foods with diarrhoea, steatorrhoea and weight loss in early adulthood.
- Mild forms may present later in life with non-specific symptoms of malaise, anaemia (including iron deficiency picture), abdominal cramps and weight loss.

Crohn's disease

- Most Common presenting symptoms are colicky abdominal pains with diarrhoea and weight loss.
- Malabsorption is an uncommon presenting symptom but often accompanies stenosing or inflammatory complications of widespread ileal disease.

Intestinal resection

- Global malabsorption may develop after small bowel resections leaving less than 50 cm of functional ileum. Water and electrolyte balance is most disordered but fat, vitamin and other nutrient absorption is also affected with lengths progressively less than 50 cm.
- Specific malabsorption may result from relatively small resection (e.g. fat and vitamin B_{12} malabsorption after terminal ileal resection, vitamin B_{12} and iron malabsorption after gastrectomy).

Whipple's disease (intestinal lipodystrophy)

- Fat malabsorption caused by intestinal infection blocking the lacteals with macrophages and bacteria.

- Presents with steatorrhoea associated with arthralgia and malaise.

Bacterial overgrowth

- Malabsorption caused by bacterial metabolism of nutrients and production of breakdown products such as CO_2 and H_2.
- Usually a result of exclusion of a loop of ileum (e.g. in Crohn's disease, postsurgery, intestinal fistulation) with consequent bacterial overgrowth, although can occur in chronically damaged or dilated bowel.

Radiation enteropathy

- Slow onset, progressive global malabsorption. Usually only if large areas of ileum affected.
- May occur many years after original radiotherapy exposure.

Chronic ischaemic enteropathy

Rare cause of malabsorption. Usually accompanied by chronic intestinal ischaemia causing 'mesenteric angina/claudication' upon eating.

Parasitic infection

Common in tropics but rare in the UK.

Investigations

- FBC, U+E, LFTs: general nutritional status.
- Trace elements (Zn, Se, Mg, Mn, Cu).
- Anti a-gliadin antibodies (serum assay for coeliac disease).
- Small bowel meal or enema: best for Crohn's disease, radiation or ischaemic enteropathy and blind loop formation.

Essential management

- Major deficiencies should be corrected by supplementation (oral or parenteral).
- Infectious causes should be excluded or (consider probiotics) treated promptly.
- Coeliac disease: gluten-free diet.
- Crohn's disease: usually requires resection of affected segment. Course of systemic steroids or immunosuppressive agents may help.
- Radiation or ischaemic malabsorption rarely responds to any medical therapy—often requires parenteral nutrition.

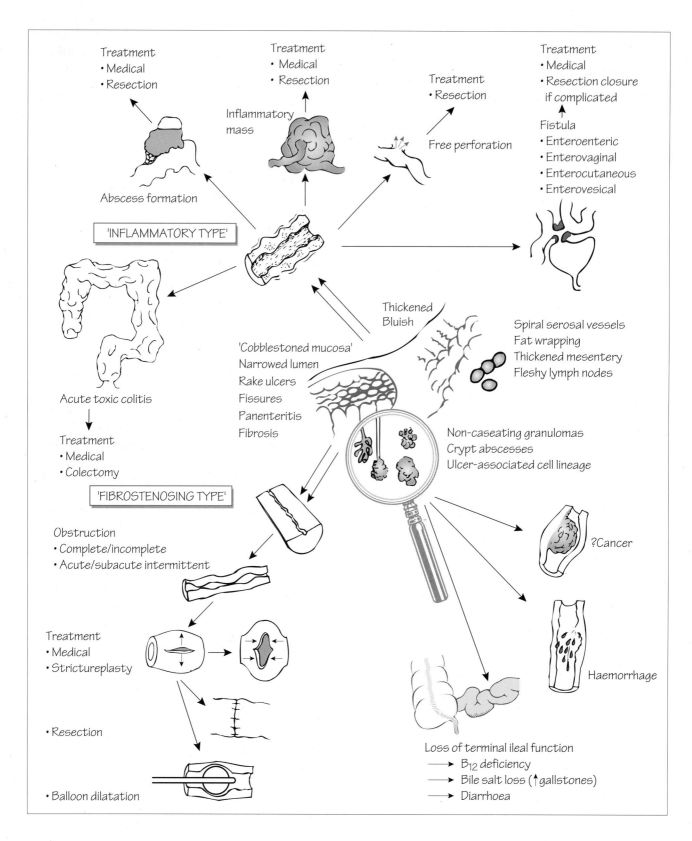

Treatment
• Medical
• Resection

Treatment
• Medical
• Resection

Inflammatory mass

Treatment
• Resection

Free perforation

Treatment
• Medical
• Resection closure
  if complicated

Fistula
• Enteroenteric
• Enterovaginal
• Enterocutaneous
• Enterovesical

Abscess formation

'INFLAMMATORY TYPE'

Thickened
Bluish

Spiral serosal vessels
Fat wrapping
Thickened mesentery
Fleshy lymph nodes

'Cobblestoned mucosa'
Narrowed lumen
Rake ulcers
Fissures
Panenteritis
Fibrosis

Acute toxic colitis

Treatment
• Medical
• Colectomy

'FIBROSTENOSING TYPE'

Non-caseating granulomas
Crypt abscesses
Ulcer-associated cell lineage

?Cancer

Obstruction
• Complete/incomplete
• Acute/subacute intermittent

Treatment
• Medical
• Strictureplasty

• Resection

Haemorrhage

• Balloon dilatation

Loss of terminal ileal function
⟶ B$_{12}$ deficiency
⟶ Bile salt loss (↑gallstones)
⟶ Diarrhoea

Definition

Crohn's disease is a chronic transmural inflammatory disorder of the alimentary tract.

Key points

- May present with acute, subacute or chronic manifestations.
- Perianal disease is common and may be the presenting feature.
- Surgery is common but never curative and should be used sparingly when necessary.

Epidemiology

Male/female 1 : 1.6. Young adults. High incidence among Europeans and Jewish people.

Aetiology

- Unknown.
- Impaired cell-mediated immunity.
- Genetic link probable but candidate genes unknown.
- No proven link to mycobacterial infection or measles virus hypersensitivity.
- Smoking associated with recurrence.

Pathology
Macroscopic

- May affect any part of the alimentary tract.
- Skip lesions in bowel (affected bowel wall and mesentery are thickened and oedematous, frequent fistulae).
- Affected bowel characteristically 'fat wrapped' by mesenteric fat.
- Perianal disease characterized by perianal induration and sepsis with fissure, sinus and fistula formation.

Histology

- Transmural inflammation in the form of lymphoid aggregates.
- Non-caseating epithelioid cell granulomas with Langhans giant cells. Regional nodes may also be involved.

Clinical features
Acute presentations (uncommon)

- RIF peritonitis (like appendicitis picture).
- Generalized peritonitis (due to free perforation).

Subacute presentations (common)

- RIF inflammatory mass (usually associated with fistulae or abscess formation).
- Widespread ileal inflammation—general ill health, malnutrition, anaemia, abdominal pain.

Chronic presentations

- Strictures—intermittent colicky abdominal pains associated with eating.

- Malabsorption (due to widespread disease often with previous resections).
- Growth retardation in children (due to chronic malnutrition and chronic inflammatory response suppressing growth).

Extraintestinal features

- Eye: episcleritis, uveitis.
- Acute phase proteins, e.g. C-reactive protein (CRP)
- Joints: arthritis.
- Skin: erythema nodosum, pyoderma gangrenosum.
- Liver: sclerosing cholangitis, cirrhosis.

Perianal disease

Fissure *in ano*, fistula *in ano*, perianal sepsis.

Investigations

- FBC: macrocytic anaemia.
- Acute phase proteins, e.g. C-reactive protein (CRP)
- Small bowel enema: narrowed terminal ileum, 'string sign' of Kantor, stricture formation, fistulae.
- Abdominal ultrasound: RIF mass, abscess formation.
- CT scan: RIF mass, abscess formation.
- Indium-labelled white-cell scan: areas of inflammation.

Essential management

Medical

- Nutritional support (enteral and parenteral feeding).
- Anti-inflammatory drugs (5Aminosaliylates, salazopyrin, steroids).
- Antibiotics (metronidazole or those for specific complicating bacterial infections).
- Immunosuppressive agents (azathioprine, methotrexate, cyclosporin A).

Surgical
For

- Complications (peritonitis, obstruction, abscess, fistula).
- Failure of medical treatment and persisting symptoms.
- Growth retardation in children.
- Principles—resect minimum necessary and conserve length where possible.

Prognosis

- Crohn's disease is a chronic problem, and recurrent episodes of active disease are common.
- 75% of patients will require surgery at some time.
- 60% of patients will require more than one operation.
- Life expectancy of Crohn's disease patients is little different from the 'normal' population.

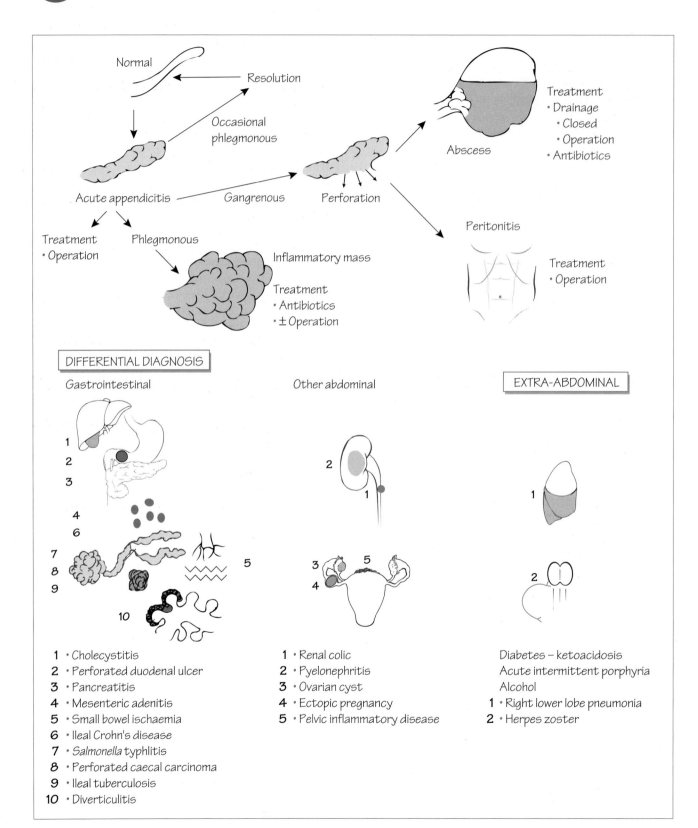

Normal

Resolution

Occasional phlegmonous

Acute appendicitis — Gangrenous — Perforation

Treatment
• Operation

Phlegmonous

Abscess

Treatment
• Drainage
  • Closed
  • Operation
• Antibiotics

Inflammatory mass

Treatment
• Antibiotics
• ± Operation

Peritonitis

Treatment
• Operation

DIFFERENTIAL DIAGNOSIS

Gastrointestinal

Other abdominal

EXTRA-ABDOMINAL

1 • Cholecystitis
2 • Perforated duodenal ulcer
3 • Pancreatitis
4 • Mesenteric adenitis
5 • Small bowel ischaemia
6 • Ileal Crohn's disease
7 • Salmonella typhlitis
8 • Perforated caecal carcinoma
9 • Ileal tuberculosis
10 • Diverticulitis

1 • Renal colic
2 • Pyelonephritis
3 • Ovarian cyst
4 • Ectopic pregnancy
5 • Pelvic inflammatory disease

Diabetes – ketoacidosis
Acute intermittent porphyria
Alcohol
1 • Right lower lobe pneumonia
2 • Herpes zoster

Definition

Acute appendicitis is an inflammation of the vermiform appendix.

Key points

- 7 out of 10 cases of RIF pain in children under 10 are non-specific and self limiting.
- The most common differential diagnosis in young women is ovarian pathology.
- RIF peritonism over 55 years should raise the suspicion of other causes.
- Cross-sectional imaging (CT) should be obtained whenever there is real concern about the differential diagnosis to prevent inappropriate surgical exploration.

Epidemiology

Most common surgical emergency in the Western world. Rare under 2 years, common in second and third decades, but can occur at any age.

Pathology

- 'Obstructive'—infection superimposed on luminal obstruction from any cause.
- 'Phlegmonous'—viral infection, lymphoid hyperplasia, ulceration, bacterial invasion without obvious cause.

Clinical features

- Periumbilical abdominal pain, nausea, vomiting.
- Localization of pain to RIF.
- Mild pyrexia.
- Patient is flushed, tachycardia, furred tongue, halitosis.
- Tender (usually with rebound) over McBurney's point.
- Right-sided pelvic tenderness on PR examination.
- Peritonitis if appendix perforated.
- Appendix mass if patient presents late.

Investigations

- Diagnosis is a clinical diagnosis, but WCC (almost always leucocytosis) and CRP (usually raised) are helpful.
- Ultrasound for appendix mass and if in doubt to rule out other pelvic pathology (e.g. ovarian cyst).
- Laparoscopy commonly used to exclude ovarian pathology prior to appendicectomy in young women.
- CT scan (helical) in elderly patients or where other causes are considered possible.

Differential diagnosis

- Mesenteric lymphadenitis in children.
- Pelvic disease in women (e.g. pelvic inflammatory disease, UTIs, ectopic pregnancy, ruptured corpus luteum cyst).
- More rarely: Crohn's disease, cholecystitis, perforated duodenal ulcer, right basal pneumonia, torsion of the right testis, diabetes mellitus in younger and middle-aged patients.
- Occasionally: perforated caecal carcinoma, sigmoid diverticulitis, caecal diverticulitis in elderly patients.

Essential management

- Acute appendicitis: appendicectomy, open or laparoscopic.
- Appendix mass: i.v. fluids, antibiotics, close observation. Then:

  If symptoms resolve: interval appendicectomy after a few months.

  If symptoms progress: urgent appendicectomy ± drainage.

Complications

- Wound infection.
- Intra-abdominal abscess (pelvic, RIF, subphrenic).
- Adhesions.
- Abdominal actinomycosis (rare!).
- Portal pyaemia.

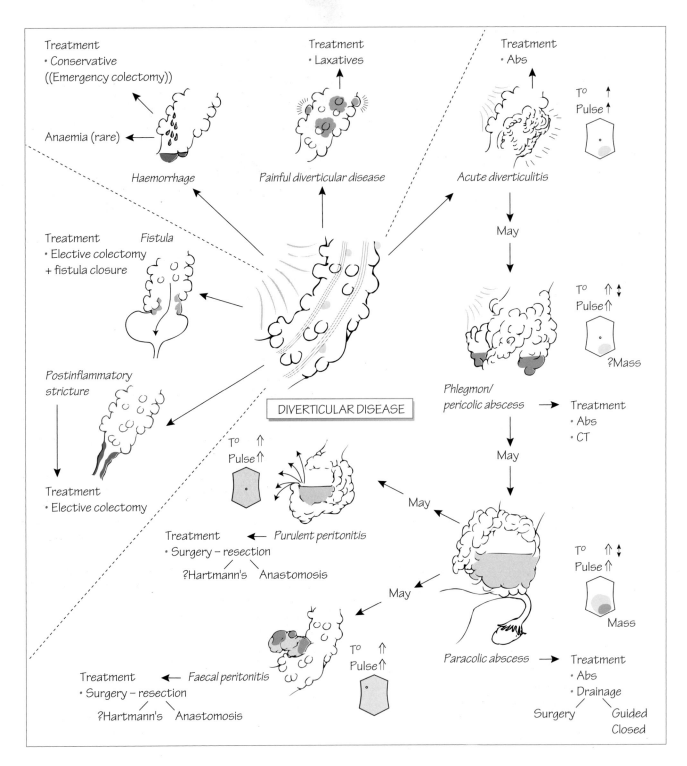

Treatment
• Conservative
((Emergency colectomy))

Anaemia (rare)

Haemorrhage

Treatment
• Laxatives

Painful diverticular disease

Treatment
• Abs

Tº ⇑
Pulse ⇑

Acute diverticulitis

May

Tº ⇑ ↕
Pulse ⇑

?Mass

Treatment   *Fistula*
• Elective colectomy
+ fistula closure

*Postinflammatory
stricture*

Treatment
• Elective colectomy

DIVERTICULAR DISEASE

*Phlegmon/
pericolic abscess* → Treatment
• Abs
• CT

May

Tº ⇑ ↕
Pulse ⇑

Mass

Tº ⇑
Pulse ⇑

May

Treatment ← *Purulent peritonitis*
• Surgery – resection

?Hartmann's   Anastomosis

May

Paracolic abscess → Treatment
• Abs
• Drainage

Surgery   Guided
Closed

Treatment ← *Faecal peritonitis*
• Surgery – resection

?Hartmann's   Anastomosis

Tº ⇑
Pulse ⇑

Definition

Diverticular disease (or diverticulosis) is a condition in which many sac-like mucosal projections (diverticula) develop in the large bowel, especially the sigmoid colon. Acute inflammation of a diverticulum causes diverticulitis.

Key points

- The majority of diverticular disease is asymptomatic.
- The majority of acute attacks are resolved by non-surgical treatment.
- Emergency surgery for complications has a high morbidity and mortality and often involves an intestinal stoma.
- Elective surgery should be reserved for recurrent proven symptoms and complications (e.g. stricture).
- 'Diverticular' strictures should be biopsied in case of underlying colon carcinoma.

Epidemiology

Male/female 1 : 1.5, peak incidence 40s and 50s onwards. High incidence in the Western world where it is found in 50% of people over 60 years.

Aetiology

- Low fibre in the diet causes an increase in intraluminal colonic pressure, resulting in herniation of the mucosa through the muscle coats of the wall of the colon.
- Weak areas in wall of colon where nutrient arteries penetrate to submucosa and mucosa.

Pathology

Macroscopic

- Diverticula mostly found in (thickened) sigmoid colon.
- Emerge between the taenia coli and may contain faecoliths.

Histological

Projections are *acquired diverticula* as they contain only mucosa, submucosa and serosa and not all layers of intestinal wall.

Clinical features

- Mostly asymptomatic.
- Painful diverticulosis: LIF pain, constipation, diarrhoea.
- Acute diverticulitis: malaise, fever, LIF pain and tenderness ± palpable mass and abdominal distension.
- Perforation: peritonitis + features of diverticulitis.
- Large bowel obstruction: absolute constipation, distension, colicky abdominal pain and vomiting.

- Fistula: to bladder (cystitis/pneumaturia/recurrent UTIs); to vagina (faecal discharge PV); to small intestine (diarrhoea).
- Lower GI bleed: painless spontaneous—distinguish from angiodysplasia.

Investigations

- Diverticulosis: barium enema (colonoscopy).
- Diverticulitis: FBC, WCC, U+E, chest X-ray, CT scan.
- ?Diverticular mass/paracolic abscess: CT scan.
- ?Perforation: plain film of abdomen, CT scan.
- ?Obstruction: gastrograffin or dilute barium enema, colonoscopy to exclude underlying malignancy.
- ?Fistula:
  colovesical—MSU, cystoscopy, barium enema;
  colovaginal—colposcopy, flexible sigmoidoscopy.
- Haemorrhage: colonoscopy, selective angiography.

Essential management

Medical

Painful or asymptomatic

High-fibre diet (fruit, vegetables, wholemeal breads, bran). Increase fluid intake.

Acute diverticulitis

- Antibiotics and bowel rest.
- Radiologically guided drainage for localized abscess.

Surgical

- Usually for complications/recurrent, proven, acute attacks or (rarely) failed medical treatment.
- Elective left colon surgery without peritonitis: resect diseased colon and rejoin the ends (primary anastomosis).
- Emergency left colon surgery with diffuse peritonitis: resect diseased segment, oversew distal bowel (i.e. upper rectum) and bring out proximal bowel as end-colostomy (Hartmann's procedure).
- Emergency left colon surgery with limited or no peritonitis: resect diseased segment and rejoin the ends (primary anastomosis) may be safe.
- Complicated left colon surgery (e.g. colovesical fistula): resection, primary anastomosis (may have defunctioning proximal stoma).

Prognosis

Diverticular disease is a 'benign' condition, but there is significant mortality and morbidity from the complications.

47 Ulcerative colitis

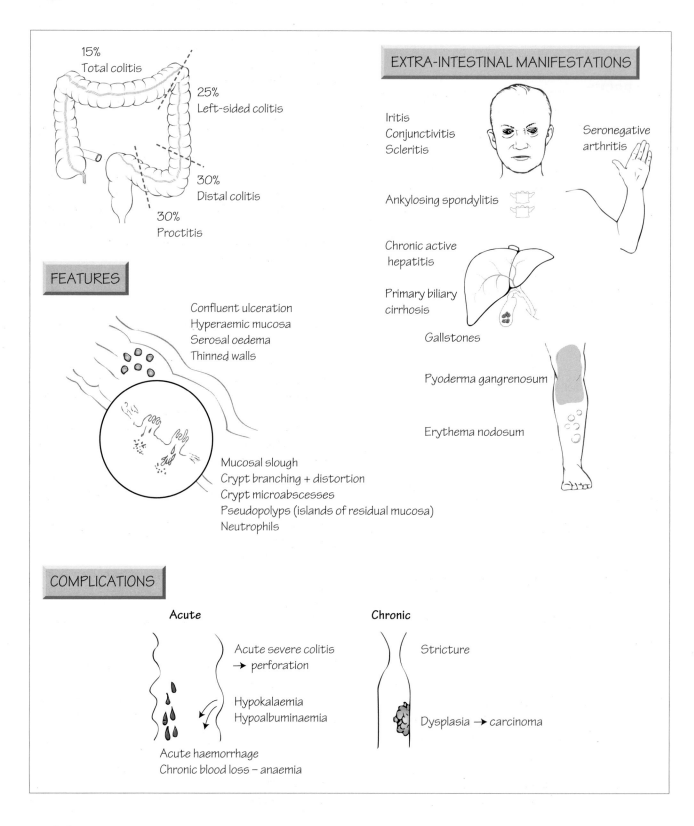

15%
Total colitis

25%
Left-sided colitis

30%
Distal colitis

30%
Proctitis

EXTRA-INTESTINAL MANIFESTATIONS

Iritis
Conjunctivitis
Scleritis

Seronegative arthritis

Ankylosing spondylitis

Chronic active hepatitis

Primary biliary cirrhosis

Gallstones

Pyoderma gangrenosum

Erythema nodosum

FEATURES

Confluent ulceration
Hyperaemic mucosa
Serosal oedema
Thinned walls

Mucosal slough
Crypt branching + distortion
Crypt microabscesses
Pseudopolyps (islands of residual mucosa)
Neutrophils

COMPLICATIONS

Acute

Acute severe colitis
→ perforation

Hypokalaemia
Hypoalbuminaemia

Acute haemorrhage
Chronic blood loss – anaemia

Chronic

Stricture

Dysplasia → carcinoma

Definition

A chronic inflammatory disorder of the colonic mucosa, usually beginning in the rectum and extending proximally to a variable extent.

Key points

- The majority of colitis is controlled by medical management —surgery is usually only required for poor control of symptoms or complications.
- Acute attacks require close scrutiny to avoid major complications.
- Long-term colitis carries a risk of colonic malignancy.
- Ileoanal pouch reconstruction offers good function in the majority of cases where surgery is required.

Epidemiology

Male/female 1 : 1.6, peak incidence 30–50 years. High incidence among relatives of patients (up to 40%) and among Europeans and Jewish people.

Aetiology

- Genetic origin: increased prevalence (10%) in relatives, associated with HLA-B27 phenotype.
- May have autoimmune basis.
- Smoking protects against relapse!

Pathology

Disease confined to colon, rectum always involved, may be 'backwash' ileitis.

Macroscopic

Only the mucosa is involved with superficial ulceration, exudation and pseudopolyposis.

Histological

Crypt abscess, inflammatory polyps and highly vascular granulation tissue. Epithelial dysplasia with longstanding disease.

Clinical features

Proctitis

- Mucus, pus and blood PR.
- Diarrhoea with urgency and frequency.

Left-sided colitis → total colitis

Symptoms of proctitis + increasing features of systemic upset, abdominal pain, anorexia, weight loss and anaemia with more extensive disease.

Extraintestinal features

Percentage involved:
- joints: arthritis (25%);
- eye: uveitis (10%);
- skin: erythema nodosum, pyoderma gangrenosum (10%);
- liver: pericholangitis, fatty liver (3%);
- blood: thromboembolic disease (rare).

Severe/fulminant disease

- 6–20 bloody bowel motions per day.
- Fever, anaemia, dehydration, electrolyte imbalance.
- Colonic dilatation/perforation—'toxic megacolon'.

Investigations

- FBC: iron deficiency anaemia.
- Stool culture: exclude infective colitis before treatment.
- Plain abdominal radiograph: colonic dilatation or air under diaphragm indicating perforation in fulminant colitis.
- Barium enema: loss of haustrations, shortened lead pipe colon.
- Sigmoidoscopy: inflamed friable mucosa, bleeds to touch.
- Colonoscopy: extent of disease at presentation, evaluation of response to treatment after exacerbations, screening of long-standing disease for dysplasia.
- Biopsy: typical histological features.

Essential management

Medical

- Basic: high-fibre diet, antidiarrhoeal agents (codeine phosphate, loperamide).
- First-line: anti-inflammatory drugs (salazopyrin, 5 amino-salicylic acid (5-ASA), corticosteroids).
- Second-line: other immunosuppressive agents (azathioprine, cyclosporin A).
- Use enemas if disease confined to rectum.
- Oral preparations for more extensive disease.
- i.v. immunosuppressives for acute exacerbations.

Surgical

Indications

- Failure of medical treatment to control chronic symptoms.
- Complications: profuse haemorrhage, perforation/acute severe colitis, risk of cancer (greater with longer disease, more aggressive onset and more extensive disease).
- Dysplasia or development of carcinoma.

Operations

- For acute attacks/complications—total colectomy, end ileostomy and preserved rectal stump.
- Electively—proctocolectomy with end (Brooke) ileostomy or proctocolectomy with preservation of anal sphincter and creation of ileoanal pouch (e.g. J-shaped pouch).

Prognosis

Ulcerative colitis is a chronic problem that requires constant surveillance unless surgery, which is drastic but curative, is performed.

Right-sided

5%

15%
Caecal

• Anaemia (bleeding)
• Weight loss
• Right iliac fossa mass (rarely small bowel obstruction)

Elective → Right hemicolectomy

Emergency → Right hemicolectomy

Left-sided

10%

20%
Sigmoid

• Altered bowel habit
• Altered blood per rectum
• 1/3 large bowel obstruction

Elective → Left/sigmoid hemicolectomy

Emergency → Hartmann's procedure

• Altered bowel habit
• Fresh blood per rectum
• Mucus per rectum
• Tenesmus
• Mass per rectum

50%
Rectal

Either → Anterior resection

→ Abdomino-perineal excision of rectum

TYPES

Polyp

Ulcer

Mass

Stricture

DUKES' STAGE

A Confined to wall

B Through bowel wall

C Involved lymph nodes (whatever the state of the primary tumour)

D Distant metastases

T1 T2 T3 T4

Mucosa
Submucosa
Musc. propria
Serosa

Definition

Colorectal carcinoma (CRC) is the occurrence of malignant lesions in the mucosa of the colon or rectum.

Key points

- Genetic factors have an important role in risk of CRC.
- Most colorectal cancers are left sided and produce symptoms of bleeding or altered bowel habit.
- Prognosis depends mainly on stage at diagnosis.
- Surgery is the only curative treatment but radiotherapy and chemotherapy are both useful adjuncts.

Epidemiology

Male/female 1.3:1, peak incidence 50+ years. Incidence has increased in Western world over last 50 years.

Aetiology

Predisposing factors in decreasing importance:
- a prior CRC or adenomatous polyps;
- hereditary polyposis syndromes;
- family history of CRC; or
- chronic active ulcerative colitis;
- diet (low in indigestible fibre, high in animal fat);
- increased faecal bile salts, selenium deficiency.

Pathology

Macroscopic

- Polypoid, ulcerating, annular, infiltrative.
- 75% of lesions are within 60 cm of the anal margin (rectum, sigmoid, left colon).
- 3% are synchronous (i.e. a second lesion will be found at the same time) and 3% are metachronous (i.e. a second lesion will be found later).

Histological

- Adenocarcinoma (10–15% are mucinous adenocarcinoma).
- Staging by Dukes' classification and TNM.
- Spread: lymphatic, haematogenous (via veins to liver), peritoneal.

Clinical features

- Anaemia—caecal cancers often present with anaemia.
- Colicky abdominal pain—tumours which are causing partial obstruction, e.g. transverse or descending colonic lesions.
- Alteration in bowel habit—either constipation or diarrhoea.
- Bleeding or passage of mucus PR.
- Tenesmus (frequent or continuous desire to defaecate)—rectal lesions.

Investigations

- Digital rectal examination and faecal occult blood.
- FBC: anaemia.
- U+E: hypokalaemia, LFTs: liver metastases.
- Sigmoidoscopy (rigid to 30 cm/flexible to 60 cm) and colonoscopy (whole colon)—see the lesion, obtain biopsy.
- Double-contrast barium enema—'apple core lesion', polyp.
- CEA is often raised in advanced disease.

Essential management

Surgery (potentially curative)

Resection of the tumour with adequate margins to include regional lymph nodes.

Procedures
- Right hemicolectomy (+/– bowel preparation) for lesions from caecum to hepatic flexure.
- Extended right hemicolectomy for lesions of the transverse colon.
- Left hemicolectomy (bowel preparation) for lesions of descending colon.
- Anterior resection for sigmoid and rectal tumours.
- Abdomino-perineal resection and colostomy for very low rectal lesions.
- Hartmann's procedure or resection with primary anastomosis for emergency surgery to left sided colon tumours.
- Resection occasionally possible for liver or lung metastases if anatomically resectable with no evidence of other disseminated disease.

Surgery/interventions (palliative)

- Open resection of the tumour (with anastomosis or stoma) for obstructing or symptomatic cancers despite metastases.
- Surgical bypass or defunctioning stoma for obstructing inoperable cancers.
- Transanal resection for inoperable rectal cancer.
- Intraluminal stents for obstructing cancers.

Other treatment

- Chemoradiotherapy may be used to shrink rectal cancers preoperatively or palliate inoperable rectal cancer.
- Adjuvant chemotherapy (5-FU ± levamisole) to reduce risk of systemic recurrence (+ve lymph nodes or presence of lymphovascular invasion).
- Adjuvant pelvic radiotherapy occasionally used to reduce risk of recurrence after rectal cancer excision with positive margins.
- Palliative chemotherapy (e.g. 5-FU) may be used to treat liver metastases or systemic disease.

Prognosis

- 5-year survival depends on staging: A, 80%; B, 60%; C, 35%; D, 5%.
- 25% 5-year survival after successful resections of liver metastases.

2 Week wait referral criteria for suspected colorectal cancer

- Rectal bleeding + increased frequency or loose stools >6 weeks
- Rectal bleeding without anal symptoms
- Increased frequency or looser stools ?6 weeks
- Rectal mass
- Right sided abdominal mass
- Iron deficiency anaemia without obvious cause

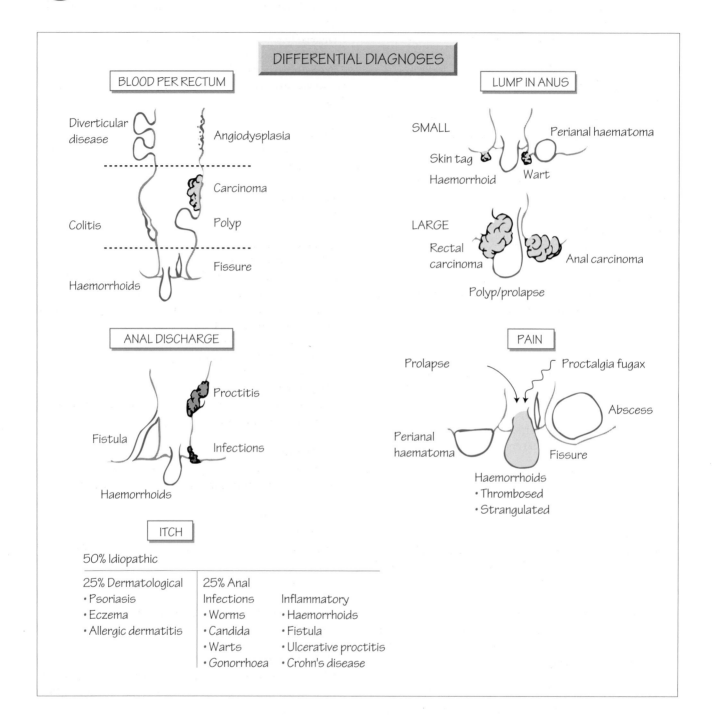

DIFFERENTIAL DIAGNOSES

BLOOD PER RECTUM

Diverticular disease — Angiodysplasia

Carcinoma

Colitis — Polyp

Fissure

Haemorrhoids

LUMP IN ANUS

SMALL — Perianal haematoma

Skin tag

Haemorrhoid — Wart

LARGE

Rectal carcinoma — Anal carcinoma

Polyp/prolapse

ANAL DISCHARGE

Proctitis

Fistula — Infections

Haemorrhoids

PAIN

Prolapse — Proctalgia fugax

Abscess

Perianal haematoma — Fissure

Haemorrhoids
• Thrombosed
• Strangulated

ITCH

50% Idiopathic

25% Dermatological	25% Anal	
• Psoriasis	Infections	Inflammatory
• Eczema	• Worms	• Haemorrhoids
• Allergic dermatitis	• Candida	• Fistula
	• Warts	• Ulcerative proctitis
	• Gonorrhoea	• Crohn's disease

Haemorrhoids ('piles')
Definition
A submucosal swelling in the anal canal consisting of a dilated venous plexus, a small artery and areolar tissue. Internal: only involves tissue of upper anal canal. External: involves tissue of lower anal canal.

Aetiology
• Increased venous pressure from straining (low-fibre diet) or altered haemodynamics (e.g. during pregnancy) causes chronic dilation of submucosal venous plexus.
• Found at the 3, 7 and 11 o'clock positions in the anal canal.

Clinical features
• First degree (1°): bleeding/itching only.
• Second degree (2°): prolapse during defaecation.
• Third degree (3°): constantly prolapsed.

Treatment

- Simple treatment—bulk laxatives and high-fibre diet.
- Bleeding internal piles—injection sclerotherapy, Barron's bands, cryosurgery.
- Prolapsing external—haemorrhoidectomy (complications: bleeding, anal stenosis).

Rectal prolapse
Definition
The protrusion from the anus to a variable degree of the rectal mucosa (partial) or rectal wall (full thickness).

Aetiology
Rectal intussusception, poor sphincter tone, chronic straining, pelvic floor injury.

Clinical features
Mucous discharge, bleeding, tenesmus, obvious prolapse.

Treatment
Stool manipulation and biofeedback, Delorme's perianal mucosal resection, abdominal rectopexy (rectum is 'hitched' up onto sacrum).

Perianal haematoma
Very painful subcutaneous haematoma caused by rupture of small blood vessel in the perianal area. Evacuation of the clot provides instant relief.

Anal fissure
Definition
Longitudinal tear in the mucosa of the anal canal, in the midline posteriorly (90%) or anteriorly (10%).

Aetiology
- 90% caused by local trauma during passage of constipated stool and potentiated by spasm of the internal anal sphincter.
- Other causes: pregnancy/delivery, Crohn's disease, sexually transmitted infections (often lateral position).

Clinical features
Exquisitely painful on passing bowel motion, small amount of bright red blood on toilet tissue, severe sphincter spasm, skin tag at distal end of tear ('sentinel pile').

Treatment
- First-line: stool softeners/bulking agents, local anaesthetic (LA) gels, GTN ointment.
- Second-line: botulinum toxin injection, lateral internal sphincterotomy.
- Examination under anaesthesia (EUA) and biopsy for atypical/suspicious abnormal fissures.

Perianal abscess
Aetiology
Focus of infection starts in anal glands ('cryptoglandular sepsis') and spreads into perianal tissues to cause:
- perianal abscess: adjacent to anal margin;
- ischiorectal abscess: in ischiorectal fossa;
- para-rectal abscess: above levator ani.

Recurrent abscesses are likely to be due to underlying fistula in ano.

Clinical features
Painful, red, tender, swollen mass ± fever, rigors, sweating, tachycardia.

Treatment
Incision and drainage, antibiotics.

Fistula *in ano*
Definition and aetiology
Abnormal communication between the perianal skin and the anal canal, established and persisting following drainage of a perianal abscess. May be associated with Crohn's disease (multiple fistulae), UC or TB.
- Low: below 50% of the external anal sphincter (EAS).
- High: crossing 50% or more of the EAS.

Clinical features
Chronic perianal discharge, external orifice of track with granulation tissue seen perianally.

Treatment
- Low: probing and laying open the track (fistulotomy).
- High: seton insertion, core removal of the fistula track.

Pilonidal sinus
Definition
A blind-ending track containing hairs in the skin of the natal cleft.

Aetiology
Movement of buttocks promotes hair migration into a (?congenital) sinus.

Clinical features
May present as: a natal cleft abscess, a discharging sinus in midline posterior to anal margin with hair protruding from orifice, natal cleft itch/pain.

Treatment
Good personal hygiene. Incision and drainage of abscesses excision of sinus network (primary closure requires asymetrical closure with flattening of natal cleft).

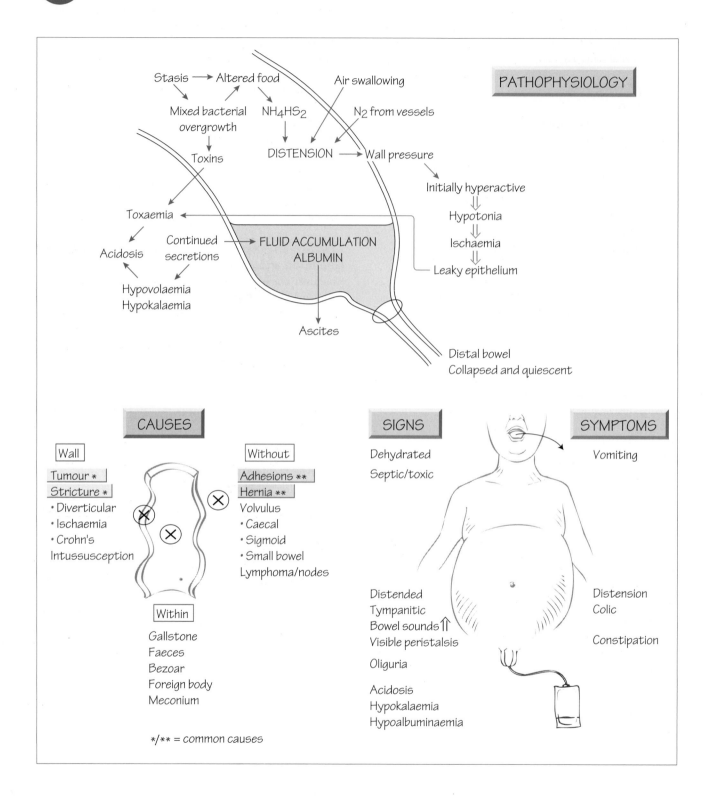

PATHOPHYSIOLOGY

Stasis → Altered food   Air swallowing

Mixed bacterial NH_4HS_2 N_2 from vessels
overgrowth

Toxins   DISTENSION → Wall pressure

Initially hyperactive
⇓
Toxaemia ←   Hypotonia
⇓
Acidosis   Continued   → FLUID ACCUMULATION   Ischaemia
secretions   ALBUMIN   ⇓
Leaky epithelium
Hypovolaemia
Hypokalaemia

Ascites

Distal bowel
Collapsed and quiescent

CAUSES

Wall

Tumour *
Stricture *
• Diverticular
• Ischaemia
• Crohn's
Intussusception

Without

Adhesions **
Hernia **
Volvulus
• Caecal
• Sigmoid
• Small bowel
Lymphoma/nodes

Within

Gallstone
Faeces
Bezoar
Foreign body
Meconium

*/** = common causes

SIGNS

Dehydrated
Septic/toxic

Distended
Tympanitic
Bowel sounds ⇑
Visible peristalsis

Oliguria

Acidosis
Hypokalaemia
Hypoalbuminaemia

SYMPTOMS

Vomiting

Distension
Colic

Constipation

Definitions

Complete intestinal obstruction indicates total blockage of the intestinal lumen, whereas *incomplete* denotes only a partial blockage. Obstruction may be *acute* (hours) or *chronic* (weeks), *simple* (*mechanical*), i.e. blood supply is not compromised, or *strangulated*, i.e. blood supply is compromised. A *closed loop obstruction* indicates that both the inlet and outlet of a bowel loop is closed off.

Key points

- Small bowel obstruction is often rapid in onset and commonly due to adhesions or hernia.
- Large bowel obstruction may be gradual or intermittent in onset, is often due to carcinoma or strictures and NEVER due to adhesions.
- All obstructed patients need fluid and electrolyte replacement.
- The cause should be sought and confirmed wherever possible prior to operation.
- Tachycardia, pyrexia and abdominal tenderness indicate the need to operate whatever the cause.

Common causes

- Extramural: adhesions, bands, volvulus, hernias (internal and external), compression by tumour (e.g. frozen pelvis).
- Intramural: inflammatory bowel disease (Crohn's disease), tumours, carcinomas, lymphomas, strictures, paralytic: (adynamic) ileus, intussusception.
- Intraluminal: faecal impaction, foreign bodies, bezoars, gallstone ileus.

Pathophysiology

- Bowel distal to obstruction collapses.
- Bowel proximal to obstruction distends and becomes hyperactive. Distension is due to swallowed air and accumulating intestinal secretions.
- The bowel wall becomes oedematous. Fluid and electrolytes accumulate in the wall and lumen (third space loss).
- Bacteria proliferate in the obstructed bowel.
- As the bowel distends, the intramural vessels become stretched and the blood supply is compromised, leading to ischaemia and necrosis.

Clinical features

- Vomiting, colicky abdominal pain, abdominal distension, absolute constipation (i.e. neither faeces nor flatus).
- Dehydration and loss of skin turgor.
- Hypotension, tachycardia.
- Abdominal distension and increased bowel sounds.
- Empty rectum on digital examination.
- Tenderness or rebound indicates peritonitis.

Investigations

- Hb, PCV: elevated due to dehydration.
- WCC: normal or slightly elevated.
- U+E: urea elevated, Na^+ and Cl^- low.
- Chest X-ray: elevated diaphragm due to abdominal distension.
- Abdominal supine X-ray:
  (a) small bowel (central loops, non-anatomical distribution, valvulae conniventes shadows cross entire width of lumen) or large bowel obstruction (peripheral distribution/haustral shadows do not cross entire width of bowel).
  (b) look for cause (gallstone, characteristic patterns of volvulus, hernias).
- Single contrast large bowel enema—?large bowel obstruction—site and cause.
- CT scan—?small bowel obstruction—site and cause, sigmoidoscopy to show site of obstruction.

Essential management

- Decompress the obstructed gut: pass nasogastric tube.
- Replace fluid and electrolyte losses: give Ringer's lactate or NaCl with K^+ supplementation.
- Monitor the patient—fluid balance chart, urinary catheter, regular temperature, pulse, respiration (TPR) chart, blood tests.
- Request investigations appropriate to likely cause.
- Relieve the obstruction surgically if:
  - underlying causes need surgical treatment (e.g. hernia, colonic carcinoma);
  - patient does not improve with conservative treatment (e.g. adhesion obstruction); or
  - there are signs of strangulation or peritonitis.

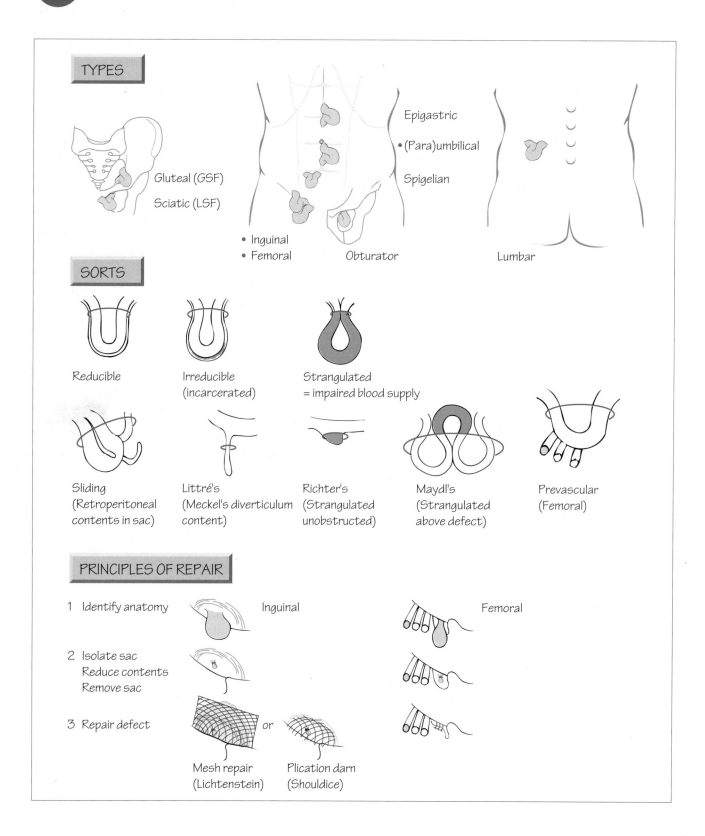

TYPES

Gluteal (GSF)

Sciatic (LSF)

Epigastric

• (Para)umbilical

Spigelian

• Inguinal
• Femoral

Obturator

Lumbar

SORTS

Reducible

Irreducible
(incarcerated)

Strangulated
= impaired blood supply

Sliding
(Retroperitoneal
contents in sac)

Littré's
(Meckel's diverticulum
content)

Richter's
(Strangulated
unobstructed)

Maydl's
(Strangulated
above defect)

Prevascular
(Femoral)

PRINCIPLES OF REPAIR

1 Identify anatomy   Inguinal   Femoral

2 Isolate sac
   Reduce contents
   Remove sac

3 Repair defect   or

Mesh repair
(Lichtenstein)

Plication darn
(Shouldice)

Definition

A hernia is the protrusion of a viscus or part of a viscus through an abnormal opening in its coverings.

Key points

- Abdominal wall hernias are common and cause many symptoms.
- Femoral hernias are more common in women than men but inguinal hernia is the most common hernia in women.
- All femoral hernias require prompt repair due to the risk of complications.
- Inguinal hernias may be repaired depending on symptoms.

Types

Common

- Umbilical/para-umbilical.
- Inguinal (direct and indirect).
- Femoral.
- Incisional.

Uncommon

- Epigastric.
- Gluteal, lumbar, obturator.

Pathophysiology

- The defect in the abdominal wall may be congenital (e.g. umbilical hernia, femoral canal) or acquired (e.g. an incision) and is lined with peritoneum (the sac).
- Raised intra-abdominal pressure further weakens the defect allowing some of the intra-abdominal contents (e.g. omentum, small bowel loop) to migrate through the opening.
- Entrapment of the contents in the sac leads to incarceration (unable to reduce contents) and possibly strangulation (blood supply to incarcerated contents is compromised).

Clinical features

- Patient presents with a lump over the site of the hernia.
- Femoral hernias are below and lateral to the pubic tubercle, they usually flatten the groin crease and are 10 times more common in women than men. 50% present as a surgical emergency due to obstructed contents and 50% of these will require a small bowel resection. Femoral hernias are irreducible.
- Inguinal hernias start off above and medial to the pubic tubercle but may descend broadly when larger, they usually accentuate the groin crease. Most are benign and have a low risk of complications.
  - (a) Indirect inguinal hernias can be controlled by digital pressure over the internal inguinal ring, may be narrow necked and are common in younger men (3% per annum present with complications).
  - (b) Direct inguinal hernias are poorly controlled by digital pressure, are often broad necked and are more common in older men (0.3% per annum strangulate).
- Incisional hernias bulge, are usually broad necked, poorly controlled by pressure and are accentuated by tensing the recti. Large, chronic incisional hernias may contain much of the small bowel and may by irreducible/unrepairable due to the 'loss of the right of abode in the abdomen' of the contents.
- True umbilical hernias are present from birth and are symmetrical defects in the umbilicus due to failure to close.
- Para-umbilical hernias develop due to an acquired defect in the periumbilical fascia.

Essential management

- Assess the hernia for: severity of symptoms, risk of complications (type, size of neck), ease of repair (size, location), likelihood of success (size, loss of right of abode).
- Assess the patient for: fitness for surgery, impact of hernia on lifestyle (job, hobbies).
- Surgical repair is usually offered in suitable patients for:
  - (a) hernias at risk of complications whatever the symptoms;
  - (b) hernias with previous symptoms of obstruction;
  - (c) hernias at low risk of complications but symptoms interfering with lifestyle, etc.

Principles of surgery

- Herniotomy: excision of the hernial sac alone for children.
- Herniorrhaphy: repairing the defect—mesh repair usual for inguinal hernias inserted via open or laparoscopic surgery.

Complications of surgery

- Haematoma (wound or scrotal).
- Acute urinary retention.
- Wound infection.
- Chronic pain.
- Testicular pain and swelling leading to testicular atrophy.
- Hernia recurrence (about 2%).

	Causes and symptoms	Cardinal symptoms and signs	Structure involved (diagnosis)		
			Gallbladder	CBD	Other
A	Presence of stone → Irritation → Contraction	Pain Nausea Vomiting Tender RUQ	Biliary colic ┊May ↓	Biliary (ductal) colic ┊May ↓	—
B	Obstruction of structure (simple)	As above + • Persistence of pain etc. • Mass RUQ (jaundice)	Mucocele ┊May ↓	Obstructive jaundice ┊May ↓	—
C	Obstruction of structure (+ infection)	As above + • Swinging fever • Tachycardia • Neutrophilia • Rigors	Empyema ┊May ↓perforate Biliary peritonitis	Cholangitis	—
D	Inflammation/ infection	As for A + • Fever • Tachycardia • Neutrophilia	Cholecystitis	(Cholangitis)	Pancreatitis

Other conditions associated with gallstones
• Gallstone ileus
• Adenocarcinoma gallbladder

CAUSES

TYPES OF GALLSTONES

Solitaire   Mulberry   Crystalline structure

Cholesterol 20%

Pigment   'Jacks'

Bile pigments 5%

Faceted   Concentric structure

Mixed 75%

Infection/ stasis   Abnormal anatomy

Diabetes mellitus
Pregnancy
Diet
Genetics
→ Cholesterol %   Lecithin %

100 0

Haematological disease
Crohn's
→ 100 Bile acids % 0

0 Sol 100

Altered bile composition

Definition

Gallstones are round, oval or faceted concretions found in the biliary tract. They contain cholesterol, calcium carbonate, calcium bilirubinate or a mixture of these elements.

Key points

- Gallstones are common and not all causes of RUQ pain with an ultrasound scan showing stones are due to gallstones.
- An episode of obstructive jaundice, deranged LFTs or acute pancreatitis or a dilated common bile duct on ultrasound scan suggests the presence of common bile duct stones.
- An attack of acute pancreatitis, cholangitis or obstructive jaundice is usually an indication for prophylactic cholecystectomy.

Epidemiology

Male/female 1 : 2. Age 40s onwards. High incidence of mixed stones in Western world. Pigment stones more common in the East.

Pathogenesis

- Cholesterol stones: imbalance in bile between cholesterol, bile salts and phospholipids, producing lithogenic bile. Associated with inflammatory bowel disease.
- Bilirubinate stones: chronic haemolysis, infection with α-glucuronidase-producing bacteria.
- Mixed stones: associated with anatomical abnormalities, stasis, previous surgery, previous infections.

Pathology

- Gallstones passing through the biliary system may cause biliary colic or pancreatitis.

- Stone obstruction at the gallbladder neck with superimposed infection leads to cholecystitis.
- Obstruction of the common bile duct (CBD) with superimposed infection leads to septic cholangitis.
- Migration of a large stone into the gut may cause intestinal obstruction (gallstone ileus).

Clinical features

- 90% of gallstones are (probably) asymptomatic.
- Biliary colic: severe colicky upper abdominal pain radiating around the right costal margin ± vomiting. Periodicity of hours, often onset at night spontaneously resolves after several hours. Differential diagnosis includes myocardial infarction, peptic ulcer exacerbation, GORD.
- 'Chronic cholecystitis': uncertain diagnosis suggested by vague, intermittent right upper abdominal pain, distension, flatulence, fatty food intolerance. May indicate recurrent mild episodes of cholecystitis. Differential diagnosis includes chronic PUD, GORD.
- Acute obstructive cholecystitis: constant right hypochondrial pain, pyrexia, nausea ± jaundice. Tender in RUQ with positive Murphy's sign. Leucocytosis. Unresolved may lead to an empyema of the gallbladder. Differential diagnosis includes myocardial infarction, basal pneumonia, pancreatitis, appendicitis, perforated peptic ulcer, pulmonary embolus.
- Cholangitis: abdominal pain, high fever/rigors, obstructive jaundice (Charcot's triad), severe RUQ tenderness. Differential diagnosis includes myocardial infarction, basal pneumonia, pancreatitis, acute hepatitis.
- Obstructive jaundice: upper abdominal pain, pale/claylike stools, dark brown urine, pruritus. May progress into cholangitis if CBD remains obstructed.
- Pancreatitis (see p. 124): central/epigastric pain, back pain, fever, tachycardia, epigastric tenderness.

Gallstone disease/2

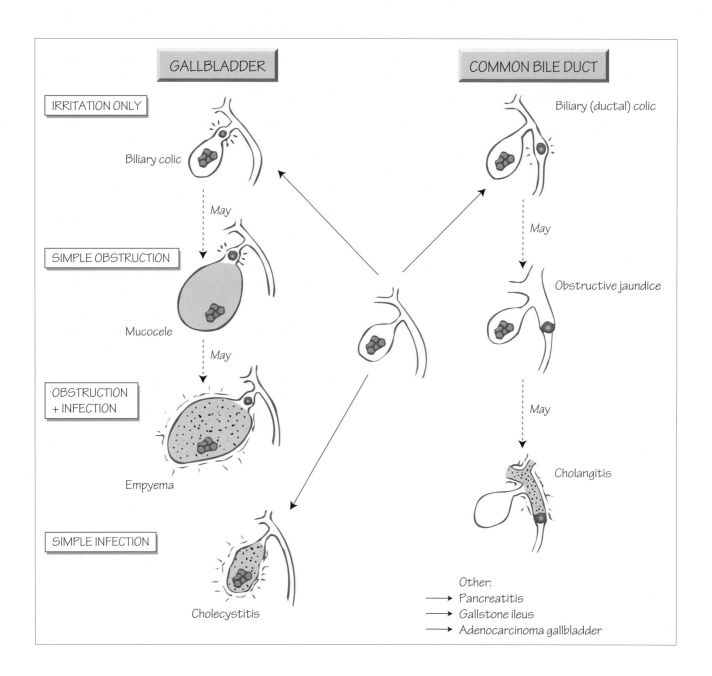

GALLBLADDER

COMMON BILE DUCT

IRRITATION ONLY

Biliary colic

Biliary (ductal) colic

May

SIMPLE OBSTRUCTION

Mucocele

May

Obstructive jaundice

May

·OBSTRUCTION + INFECTION

Empyema

May

Cholangitis

SIMPLE INFECTION

Cholecystitis

Other:
→ Pancreatitis
→ Gallstone ileus
→ Adenocarcinoma gallbladder

Investigations

• FBC: acute inflammatory complications, picture of haemolytic anaemias underlying.
• U+E.
• LFTs: obstructive jaundice pattern.
• Plain X-ray of the abdomen shows only 10% of gallstones.
• Ultrasound: 90% of gallstones will be detected on ultrasound examination. Assesses CBD size and possible presence of CBD stones.
• Rarely are other investigations, such as oral cholecystography, intravenous cholangiography or HIDA scanning, required (ultrasound impossible, e.g. obesity).
• Endoscopic retrograde cholangiopancreatography (ERCP)—suspected or proven CBD stones. Allows stones removal or stent to be placed to bypass any risk of obstruction from the stones.
• OGD: to exclude PUD as a cause for uncomplicated disease symptoms.

Essential management

• Asymptomatic: no treatment required unless diabetic or undergoing major immunosuppression (risk factors for cholecystitis).
• Biliary colic: elective cholecystectomy, now usually performed laparoscopically, for classic symptoms with ultrasound-proven gallstones.
• Chronic cholecystitis: elective laparoscopic cholecystectomy only if no evidence of PUD or other causes for symptoms.
• Acute cholecystitis: i.v. fluids, antibiotics, early or interval cholecystectomy.
• Empyema: percutaneous (ultrasound- or CT-guided) drainage of the gallbladder and interval cholecystectomy.
• Ascending cholangitis: i.v. fluids, antibiotics, ductal drainage (now usually by ERCP, sphincterotomy and extraction of stones).

Complications of cholecystectomy

• Leakage of bile from cystic duct or gallbladder bed (percutaneous drainage).
• Jaundice due to retained ductal stones. (Retained stones can be treated by ERCP or if a T-tube is in place by extraction with a Dormia basket down the T-tube track (Burhenne manoeuvre).)
• Bleeding from cystic artery or gallbladder bed (may require re-operation).
• Injury to the CBD (usually requires major reconstructive surgery).

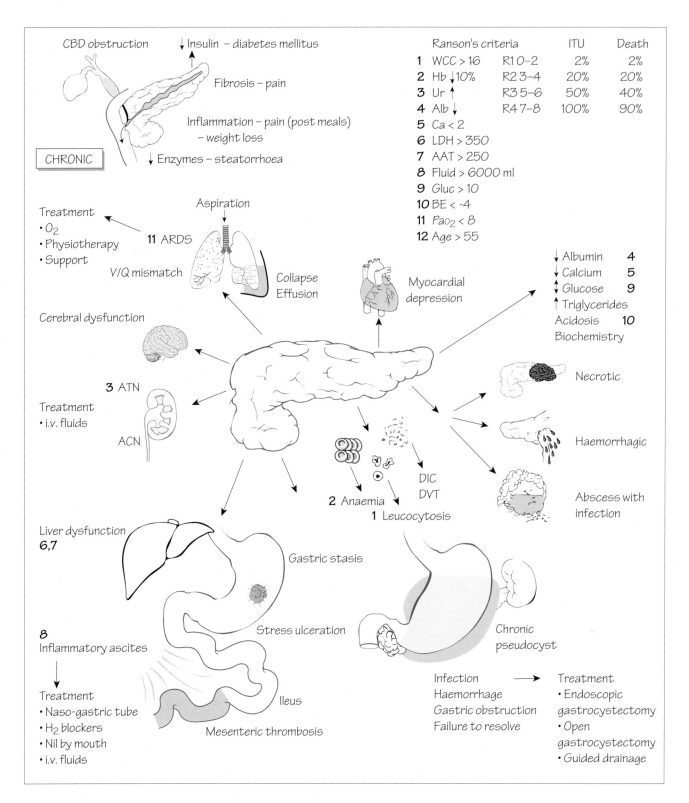

CBD obstruction   ↓ Insulin – diabetes mellitus

Fibrosis – pain

Inflammation – pain (post meals)
– weight loss

CHRONIC

↓ Enzymes – steatorrhoea

Ranson's criteria		ITU	Death
1 WCC > 16	R1 0–2	2%	2%
2 Hb ↓10%	R2 3–4	20%	20%
3 Ur ↑	R3 5–6	50%	40%
4 Alb ↓	R4 7–8	100%	90%
5 Ca < 2			
6 LDH > 350			
7 AAT > 250			
8 Fluid > 6000 ml			
9 Gluc > 10			
10 BE < -4			
11 Pao₂ < 8			
12 Age > 55			

Treatment
• O₂
• Physiotherapy
• Support

Aspiration

11 ARDS

V/Q mismatch

Collapse
Effusion

Myocardial
depression

↓ Albumin   4
↓ Calcium   5
↕ Glucose   9
↑ Triglycerides
Acidosis   10
Biochemistry

Cerebral dysfunction

3 ATN

Treatment
• i.v. fluids

ACN

Necrotic

Haemorrhagic

Abscess with
infection

2 Anaemia

DIC
DVT

1 Leucocytosis

Liver dysfunction
6,7

Gastric stasis

Stress ulceration

Chronic
pseudocyst

8
Inflammatory ascites

Treatment
• Naso-gastric tube
• H₂ blockers
• Nil by mouth
• i.v. fluids

Ileus

Mesenteric thrombosis

Infection   →   Treatment
Haemorrhage   • Endoscopic
Gastric obstruction   gastrocystectomy
Failure to resolve • Open
                    gastrocystectomy
                    • Guided drainage

Definition

An inflammatory condition of the exocrine pancreas that results from injury to the acinar cells. It may be acute or chronic.

Key points

- Most pancreatitis is mild and spontaneously resolves.
- All patients should have a cause sought by imaging and the severity assessed by recognized criteria.
- A normal or mildly elevated serum amylase does NOT exclude pancreatitis.
- Severe or complicated pancreatitis may worsen rapidly and require ICU support.
- Surgery has little place other than to treat severe complications.

Aetiology

- Gallstones and alcohol abuse account for 95% of cases of acute pancreatitis.
- Other causes include: idiopathic, congenital structural abnormalities, drugs, viral infections, hypercalcaemia, hypothermia, hyperlipidaemia and trauma.

Pathology

Acute

- Mild injury: acinar (exocrine) cell damage with enzymatic spillage, inflammatory cascade activation and localized oedema. Local exudate may also lead to increased serum levels of pancreatic enzymes (amylase, lipase, colipase).
- Moderate injury: increasing local inflammation leads to intrapancreatic bleeding, fluid collections and spreading local oedema involving the mesentery and retroperitoneum. Activation of the systemic inflammatory response leads to progressive involvement of other organs.
- Severe injury: progressive pancreatic destruction leads to necrosis, profound localized bleeding and fluid collections around the pancreas. Spread to local structures and the peritoneal cavity may result in mesenteric infarction, peritonitis and intra-abdominal fat 'saponification'.

A persisting accumulation of inflammatory fluid, usually in the lesser sac, is a pseudocyst, i.e. does not have an epithelial lining.

Chronic

Recurrent episodes of acute inflammation lead to progressive destruction of acinar cells with healing by fibrosis. Incidental islet cell damage may lead to endocrine gland failure.

Clinical features

- Mild/moderate pancreatitis: constant upper abdominal pain radiating to back, nausea, vomiting, pyrexia, tachycardia ± jaundice.

- Severe/necrotizing pancreatitis: severe upper abdominal pain, signs of hypovolaemic shock, respiratory and renal impairment, silent abdomen, retroperitoneal bleeding with flank and umbilical bruising (Grey Turner's and Cullen's signs).

Essential management

- Attempt to confirm diagnosis: (serum amylase > 1000 iµ diagnostic— may be clinical diagnosis).
- Assess disease severity (Imrie/Ranson criteria).
  Severe is 3+ of the following: WBC > 16×10^9/l, Pao_2 < 7.98 kPa, B glucose > 11.2 mmol/l, LDH > 350 IU/l, SGOT > 250 IU/l, PCV fall > 10%, urea > 1.8, Ca^{2+} < 2.0 mmol/l.
- Resuscitate the patient:
  Mild/moderate disease: i.v. fluids, analgesia, monitor progress with pulse, BP, temperature.
  Severe pancreatitis: full resuscitation in ICU with invasive monitoring.
- Establish the cause: ultrasound to look for gallstones.

Further management

- No proven use for routine nasogastric tube or antibiotics.
- ?Vitamin supplements and sedatives if alcoholic cause.
- Proven CBD gallstones may require urgent ERCP.
- Failure to respond to treatment or uncertain diagnosis warrants abdominal CT scan.
- Suspected/proven infection of necrotic pancreas— antibiotics ± surgical débridement.

Complications—acute pancreatitis

Acute

- Pancreatic abscess: usually necrotic pancreas present.
- Intra-abdominal sepsis.
- Necrosis of the transverse colon.
- Respiratory (ARDS) or renal (ATN) failure.
- Pancreatic haemorrhage.

Subacute/chronic

- Pseudocyst formation: may need to be drained internally or externally.
- Chronic pancreatitis.

Chronic pancreatitis

- Usually caused by chronic alcohol abuse.
- Presents with intractable abdominal pain and evidence of exocrine pancreatic failure (steatorrhoea) and eventually diabetes as well.
- Medical treatment is with analgesia and exocrine pancreatic enzyme replacement. Surgical treatment is by drainage of dilated pancreatic ducts or excision of the pancreas in some cases.

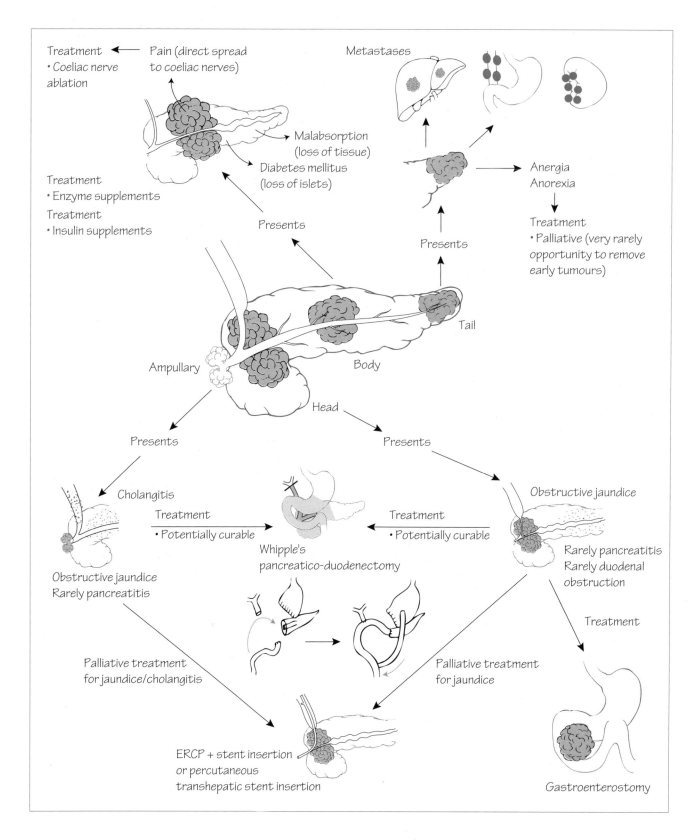

Treatment
• Coeliac nerve ablation

Pain (direct spread to coeliac nerves)

Metastases

Malabsorption (loss of tissue)

Diabetes mellitus (loss of islets)

Treatment
• Enzyme supplements

Treatment
• Insulin supplements

Presents

Anergia
Anorexia

Treatment
• Palliative (very rarely opportunity to remove early tumours)

Presents

Tail

Body

Ampullary

Head

Presents

Presents

Cholangitis

Treatment
• Potentially curable

Whipple's pancreatico-duodenectomy

Treatment
• Potentially curable

Obstructive jaundice

Obstructive jaundice
Rarely pancreatitis

Rarely pancreatitis
Rarely duodenal obstruction

Treatment

Palliative treatment for jaundice/cholangitis

Palliative treatment for jaundice

ERCP + stent insertion or percutaneous transhepatic stent insertion

Gastroenterostomy

Definitions

Pancreatic adenocarcinoma is a malignant lesion of the head, body or tail of the pancreas. *Periampullary carcinomas* arise around the ampulla of Vater and include tumours arising from the pancreas, duodenum, distal bile duct and the ampulla itself. *Endocrine pancreatic tumours* cause a variety of syndromes secondary to the secretion of active peptides.

Key points

- Most pancreatic cancer is not surgically curable.
- New, chronic back pain and vague symptoms may be the only presenting feature.
- The best prognosis is for true periampullary cancers.
- Good palliation of jaundice is possible without surgery.

Epidemiology

Male/female 2 : 1, peak incidence 50–70 years. Incidence of pancreatic carcinoma is increasing in the Western world.

Aetiology

Predisposing factors: smoking, diabetes, chronic pancreatitis.

Pathology

- Site: 55% involve head of pancreas, 25% body, 15% tail, 5% periampullary region.
- Macroscopic: growth is hard and infiltrating.
- Histology: 90% ductal carcinoma, 7% acinar cell carcinoma, 2% cystic carcinoma, 1% connective tissue origins.
- Spread: lymphatics to peritoneum and regional nodes, via bloodstream to liver and lung. Metastases often present at time of diagnosis.

Clinical features

- Head or periampullary: painless, progressive jaundice with a palpable gallbladder (Courvoisier's law: a palpable gallbladder in the presence of jaundice is unlikely to be due to gallstones).
- Occasionally duodenal obstruction causing vomiting.
- Body: back pain, anorexia, weight loss, steatorrhoea.
- Tail: often presents with metastases, malignant ascites or unexplained anaemia.

Investigations

- Ultrasound: may see mass in head of pancreas and distended biliary tree, facilitates needle biopsy.
- CT scan: demonstrates tumour mass, facilitates biopsy, assess involvement of surrounding structures and local lymph node spread.
- ERCP: very accurate in making diagnosis; obtain specimen or shed cells for cytology and stent may be placed to relieve jaundice.
- Barium meal: widening of the duodenal loop with medial filling defect, the reversed '3' sign.

Essential management

Palliation

- Pancreatic adenocarcinoma is usually incurable at time of diagnosis.
- Jaundice can be relieved by placing a stent through the tumour either transhepatically or via ERCP.
- Duodenal obstruction may be relieved by gastrojejunostomy.
- Pain may be helped with a coeliac axis block.

Curative treatment

Rarely surgical (Whipple's) resection of small tumours of the head of the pancreas is curative if lymph nodes are not involved.

Prognosis

- 90% of patients with pancreatic adenocarcinoma are dead within 12 months of diagnosis.
- It is important to obtain histology from tumours around the head of the pancreas as the prognosis from non-pancreatic peri-ampullary cancers is considerably better (50% 5-year survival) following resection.

2 Week wait referral criteria for suspected upper GI cancer

- New onset dysphagia (any age)
- Dyspepsia + weight loss/anaemia/vomitting
- Dyspepsia + FHx/Barrett's oesophagus/previous peptic ulcer surgery/atrophic gastritis/pernicious anaemia
- New dyspepsia > 55 years
- Jaundice
- Upper abdominal mass

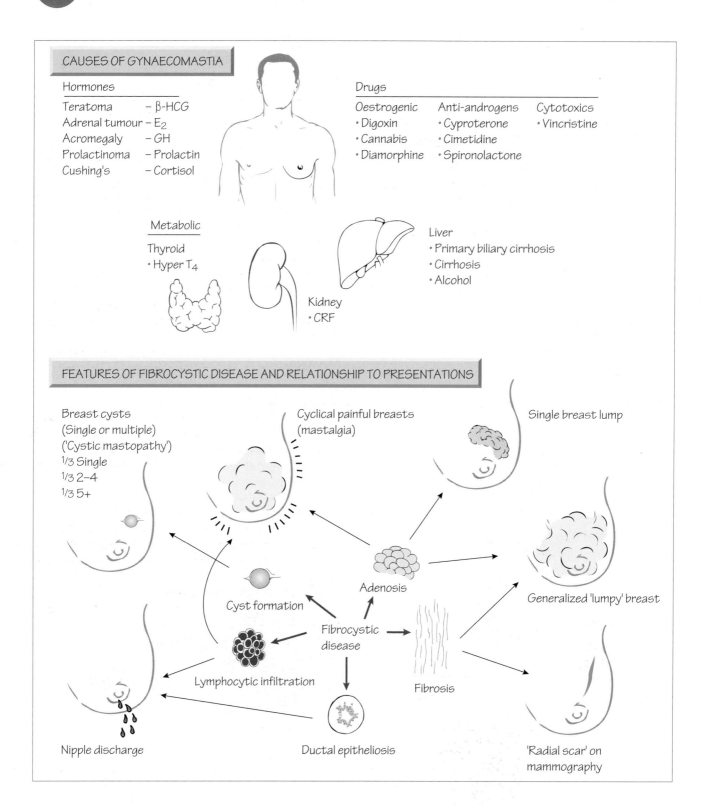

CAUSES OF GYNAECOMASTIA

Hormones

Teratoma	– β-HCG
Adrenal tumour	– E_2
Acromegaly	– GH
Prolactinoma	– Prolactin
Cushing's	– Cortisol

Drugs

Oestrogenic	Anti-androgens	Cytotoxics
• Digoxin	• Cyproterone	• Vincristine
• Cannabis	• Cimetidine	
• Diamorphine	• Spironolactone	

Metabolic

Thyroid
• Hyper T_4

Kidney
• CRF

Liver
• Primary biliary cirrhosis
• Cirrhosis
• Alcohol

FEATURES OF FIBROCYSTIC DISEASE AND RELATIONSHIP TO PRESENTATIONS

Breast cysts
(Single or multiple)
('Cystic mastopathy')
1/3 Single
1/3 2–4
1/3 5+

Cyclical painful breasts
(mastalgia)

Single breast lump

Cyst formation

Adenosis

Generalized 'lumpy' breast

Fibrocystic disease

Lymphocytic infiltration

Fibrosis

Nipple discharge

Ductal epitheliosis

'Radial scar' on mammography

ANDI

Definition

Abnormalities of the **N**ormal **D**evelopment and **I**nvolution of the breast—a broad term covering benign conditions many of which have overlapping features.

Key points

- Any breast lump should be evaluated by triple assessment for risk of malignancy whatever the likely diagnosis.
- ANDI disorders are common in younger, premenopausal women and often cause considerable anxiety.
- Gynaecomastia is usually physiological but often needs to be investigated for hormonal causes.

Abnormalities of development

Fibroadenoma

- Benign breast lump caused by overgrowth of single breast lobule. Manifests as one or more firm, mobile, painless lumps usually in women under 30 years.
- Investigation: 'triple assessment' (clinical/radiological/cytological) (see p. 121).
- Treatment:
  age < 30 years either observe or excise if worried;
  age > 30 years consider excision to exclude malignancy.

Abnormalities of cycles

Fibrocystic disease

- Usually presents age 25–45 years. May present as breast pain, tenderness, breast lump(s), breast cyst(s), especially during the second half of the menstrual cycle.
- Investigation: 'triple assessment' of all lumps.
- Treatment: patient reassurance, analgesics, γ-linoleic acid, hormone manipulation, cyst aspiration, excision of persistent localized masses after aspiration. Avoid xanthine-containing substances (coffee).

Abnormalities of involution

Breast cyst

- May be single or multiple. Firm, round discrete lump(s).
- Investigation: aspiration ± mammography. Triple assessment for any discrete associated lumps.

- Treatment: reassurance, aspiration (repeated), hormone manipulation.

Other benign conditions

Breast abscess

- Usually infection of the pregnant or lactating breast with *Staphylococcus aureus* (puerperal infection). Patient presents with redness, swelling, heat and pain in the breast. Chronic/recurrent sepsis associated with smoking and ductal ectasia with mixed anaerobic infection.
- Treatment: puerperal sepsis is with antibiotics (flucloxacillin) initially but, if an abscess develops, repeated aspiration or occasionally incision and drainage will be required. Lactation/breast feeding does not need to be suppressed while the abscess is being treated; chronic sepsis treat with metronidazole and recurrent aspirations if necessary.

Mammary duct ectasia

- Dilated subareolar ducts are filled with cellular debris which causes a periductal inflammatory response. Associated with smoking and recurrent non-lactational abscesses. The usual presentation is a green nipple multifocal ductal discharge and a subareolar lump.
- Treatment is by subareolar excision of the involved ducts if troublesome symptoms persist or the diagnosis is unsure.

Duct papilloma

- Small papillomas arise in the major breast ducts. They cause a bloody or serous nipple discharge usually from one duct.
- Treatment is usually by excision of the affected duct by microdochectomy if the symptoms persist.

Fat necrosis

- A fibrous scar in the breast tissue caused by injury, haematoma and necrosis of breast fat with subsequent scarring. History of trauma to the breast in 50% of cases. May be associated with superficial ecchymoses. Histology: periductal cellular infiltrate and fibrosis.
- Investigation: triple assessment.
- Treatment: surgical excision if mass fails to resolve or there is concern to exclude malignancy.

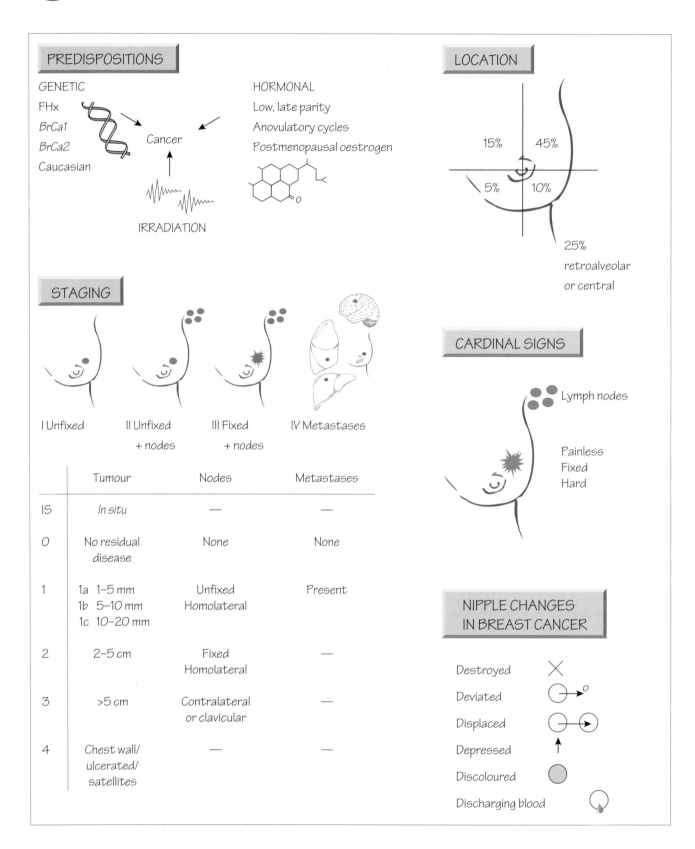

PREDISPOSITIONS

GENETIC
FHx
BrCa1
BrCa2
Caucasian

Cancer

IRRADIATION

HORMONAL
Low, late parity
Anovulatory cycles
Postmenopausal oestrogen

LOCATION

15%   45%
5%   10%

25%
retroalveolar
or central

STAGING

I Unfixed   II Unfixed   III Fixed   IV Metastases
             + nodes   + nodes

	Tumour	Nodes	Metastases
IS	In situ	—	—
0	No residual disease	None	None
1	1a 1–5 mm 1b 5–10 mm 1c 10–20 mm	Unfixed Homolateral	Present
2	2–5 cm	Fixed Homolateral	—
3	>5 cm	Contralateral or clavicular	—
4	Chest wall/ ulcerated/ satellites	—	—

CARDINAL SIGNS

Lymph nodes

Painless
Fixed
Hard

NIPPLE CHANGES IN BREAST CANCER

Destroyed
Deviated
Displaced
Depressed
Discoloured
Discharging blood

Definition

Malignant lesion of (predominantly) the female breast.

Key points

- All breast lumps require triple assessment.
- Early breast cancer can be effectively treated in many cases.
- Early breast cancer treatment is aimed at local control/lymph node treatment and prevention of systemic relapse.
- Treatment of late breast cancer is usually palliative and mostly medical.

Epidemiology

Male/female 1 : 100. Any age (usually > 30 years). High incidence in Western world and in white population more than black population.

Aetiology

Predisposing factors:
- strong family history of breast cancer (genetic factors);
- early menarche and late menopause, especially in nulliparous women;
- social class I and II.

Pathology

- Histology: adenocarcinomas arising from the glandular epithelium. Common types are invasive ductal (90%) or lobular (10%) carcinoma. *Paget's disease* is ductal carcinoma involving the nipple.
- Spread: lymphatics, vascular invasion, direct extension; spreads to lung, liver, bone, brain, adrenal, ovary.
- Staging: TNM classification—important for treatment and prognosis.

Clinical features

- Palpable, hard, irregular, fixed breast lump, usually painless.
- Nipple retraction and skin dimpling.
- Nipple eczema in Paget's disease.
- *Peau d'orange* (cutaneous oedema secondary to lymphatic obstruction).
- Palpable axillary nodes.

Investigations

- Triple assessment: clinical/radiological/cytological.
- Radiological assessment: mammography (ultrasound in young women with dense or large breasts). Features on mammography: irregular, spiculated, radio-opaque mass with microcalcification.
- Cytological assessment: FNAC or core biopsy.
- Breast biopsy: excision biopsy occasionally required for diagnosis.
- Staging investigations for proven carcinoma:

all: chest X-ray, FBC, serum alkaline phosphatase, γ-glutamyl transpeptidase, serum calcium—(suggest liver or bone metastases);
if clinically indicated: isotope bone scan, ultrasound scan of liver, brain CT scan.
- Breast tissue for hormone receptor status (ER± PR±, HER2 ±), important for treatment and prognosis.

Essential management

Early breast cancer

(No evidence of distant spread at time of diagnosis.)
- Local treatment is usually either:
  lumpectomy + radiotherapy to breast; or
  simple mastectomy.
- Management of axillary lymph nodes is essential in cases of invasive cancer (for staging, prognosis and treatment) usually either:
  axillary dissection and removal or axillary sampling and selective radiotherapy to axilla. Sentinel node biipsy increasingly used to determine if axiallary clearance or radiotherapy required.
- Prevention of systemic spread is usually either:
  hormonal therapy (e.g. tamoxifen or aromatase inhibitor); or adjuvant chemotherapy (anthraclines or cyclophosphamide, methotrexate, 5-FU) if high risk (positive lymph nodes, bad histological features).
- Prognosis depends on lymph nodes status, tumour size and histological grade: overall 80% 10-year survival rate.

Late breast cancer

(Distant spread at time of diagnosis.)
- Local treatment is directed at controlling local recurrence lumpectomy/mastectomy/radiotherapy.
- Distant metastases: radiotherapy to relieve pain from bony metastases, hormone treatment (tamoxifen, aromatase inhibitors, fulvestrant) if ER positive. Chemotherapy (anthraclines or taxanes or biological agents (herseptin) if HER2 positive.
- Prognosis: poor, only 30–40% respond to treatment with mean survival of 2 years, by which time the non-responders have usually died.

2 Week wait referral criteria for suspected breast cancer

- Discrete lump > 30 years
- Breast ulceration
- Breast skin nodules
- Breast skin distortion
- Nipple eczema
- Recent nipple retraction/distortion

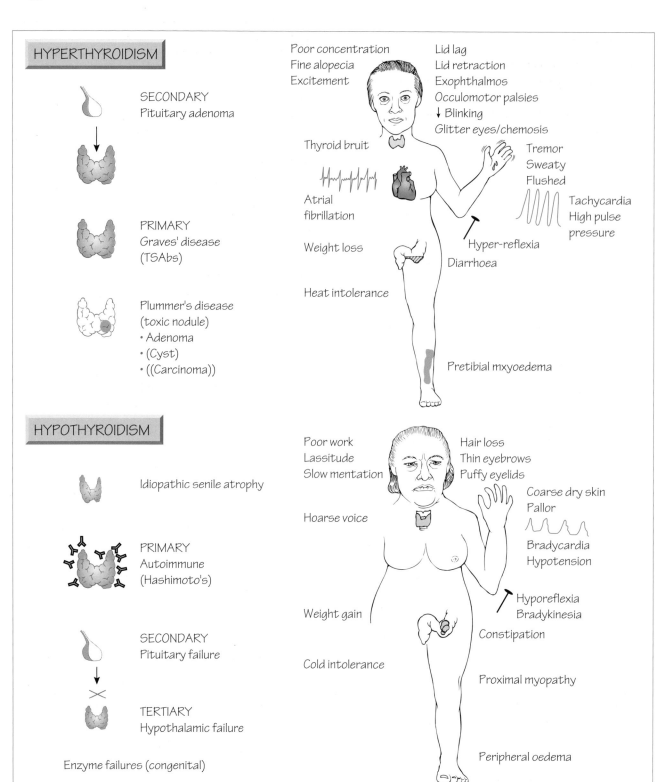

HYPERTHYROIDISM

SECONDARY
Pituitary adenoma

PRIMARY
Graves' disease
(TSAbs)

Plummer's disease
(toxic nodule)
• Adenoma
• (Cyst)
• ((Carcinoma))

Poor concentration
Fine alopecia
Excitement

Lid lag
Lid retraction
Exophthalmos
Occulomotor palsies
↓ Blinking
Glitter eyes/chemosis

Thyroid bruit

Atrial
fibrillation

Weight loss

Heat intolerance

Tremor
Sweaty
Flushed

Tachycardia
High pulse
pressure

Hyper-reflexia

Diarrhoea

Pretibial mxyoedema

HYPOTHYROIDISM

Idiopathic senile atrophy

PRIMARY
Autoimmune
(Hashimoto's)

SECONDARY
Pituitary failure

TERTIARY
Hypothalamic failure

Enzyme failures (congenital)

Poor work
Lassitude
Slow mentation

Hoarse voice

Weight gain

Cold intolerance

Hair loss
Thin eyebrows
Puffy eyelids

Coarse dry skin
Pallor

Bradycardia
Hypotension

Hyporeflexia
Bradykinesia

Constipation

Proximal myopathy

Peripheral oedema

Definition

A *goitre* is an enlargement of the thyroid gland from any cause.

Key points

- Toxic goitres are rarely malignant.
- All solitary nodules need investigation to exclude carcinoma.
- Surgery is rarely necessary in autoimmune or inflammatory thyroid disease.

Common causes

- Physiological: gland increases in size as a result of increased demand for thyroid hormone at puberty and during pregnancy.
- Iodine deficiency (endemic): deficiency of iodine results in decreased T_4 levels and increased TSH stimulation leading to a diffuse goitre.
- Primary hyperthyroidism (Graves' disease): goitre and thyrotoxicosis due to circulating immunoglobulin LATS.
- Adenomatous (nodular) goitre: benign hyperplasia of the thyroid gland.
- Thyroiditis: autoimmune (Hashimoto's); subacute (de Quervain's); Riedel's (struma).
- Thyroid malignancies.

Clinical features

Hyperthyroidism

Symptoms

- Heat intolerance and excessive sweating.
- Increased appetite, weight loss, diarrhoea.
- Anxiety, tiredness, palpitations.
- Oligomenorrhoea.

Signs

- Goitre.
- Exophthalmos, lid lag and retraction.
- Warm moist palms, tremor.
- Atrial fibrillation.
- Pretibial myxoedema.

Hypothyroidism

Symptoms

- Cold intolerance, decreased sweating.
- Hoarseness.
- Weight increase, constipation.
- Slow cerebration, tiredness.
- Muscle pains.

Signs

- Pale/yellow skin, dry, thickened skin, thin hair.
- Periorbital puffiness, loss of outer third of eyebrow.
- Dementia, nerve deafness, hyporeflexia.
- Slow pulse, large tongue, peripheral oedema.

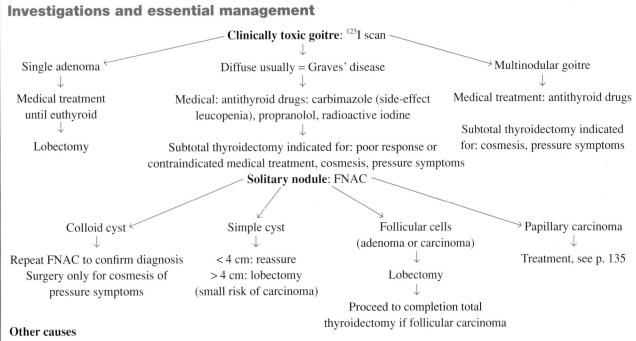

Investigations and essential management

Clinically toxic goitre: ^{123}I scan

Single adenoma
↓
Medical treatment until euthyroid
↓
Lobectomy

Diffuse usually = Graves' disease
↓
Medical: antithyroid drugs: carbimazole (side-effect leucopenia), propranolol, radioactive iodine
↓
Subtotal thyroidectomy indicated for: poor response or contraindicated medical treatment, cosmesis, pressure symptoms

Multinodular goitre
↓
Medical treatment: antithyroid drugs

Subtotal thyroidectomy indicated for: cosmesis, pressure symptoms

Solitary nodule: FNAC

Colloid cyst
↓
Repeat FNAC to confirm diagnosis
Surgery only for cosmesis of pressure symptoms

Simple cyst
↓
< 4 cm: reassure
> 4 cm: lobectomy
(small risk of carcinoma)

Follicular cells (adenoma or carcinoma)
↓
Lobectomy
↓
Proceed to completion total thyroidectomy if follicular carcinoma

Papillary carcinoma
↓
Treatment, see p. 135

Other causes

- Physiological: reassurance.
- I_2 deficiency (endemic): supplemental iodine in the diet.
- Thyroiditis.
- Autoimmune (Hashimoto's): anti-inflammatories, thyroid replacement therapy if becomes hypothyroid.
- Subacute (de Quervain's): simple analgesia, sometimes steroids.
- Riedel's (struma): resection only for compression symptoms.

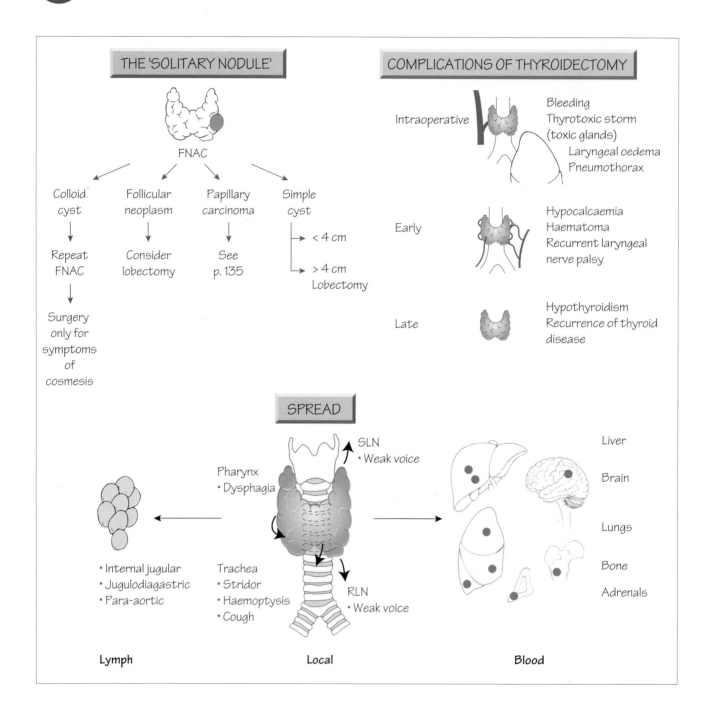

THE 'SOLITARY NODULE'

FNAC

Colloid cyst → Repeat FNAC → Surgery only for symptoms of cosmesis

Follicular neoplasm → Consider lobectomy

Papillary carcinoma → See p. 135

Simple cyst → < 4 cm / > 4 cm Lobectomy

COMPLICATIONS OF THYROIDECTOMY

Intraoperative — Bleeding, Thyrotoxic storm (toxic glands), Laryngeal oedema, Pneumothorax

Early — Hypocalcaemia, Haematoma, Recurrent laryngeal nerve palsy

Late — Hypothyroidism, Recurrence of thyroid disease

SPREAD

SLN • Weak voice

Pharynx • Dysphagia

RLN • Weak voice

• Internal jugular
• Jugulodiagastric
• Para-aortic

Trachea
• Stridor
• Haemoptysis
• Cough

Liver
Brain
Lungs
Bone
Adrenals

Lymph   **Local**   **Blood**

Definition

Malignant lesions of the thyroid gland.

Key points

- Many thyroid tumours are tumours of young adults.
- Isolated thyroid lumps should always be investigated to confirm a cause.
- The prognosis is often good with surgical resection and medical adjuvant treatment.

Epidemiology

Male/female 1 : 2. Peak incidence depends on histology (papillary: young adults; follicular: middle age; anaplastic: elderly; medullary: any age).

Pathology

Histology of thyroid malignancies.

Type	(% of total)	Cell of origin	Differentiation	Spread
Papillary	(60%)	Epithelial	Well	Lymphatic
Follicular	(25%)	Epithelial	Well	Haematogenous
Anaplastic	(10%)	Epithelial	Poor	Direct, lymphatic and haematogenous
Medullary	(5%)	Parafollicular	Moderate	Lymphatic and haematogenous

Essential management

Papillary

- Surgery: total thyroidectomy and removal of involved lymph nodes.
- Adjunctive treatment: L-thyroxine postoperatively to suppress TSH production (which stimulates papillary tumour growth).
- Prognosis: excellent.

Follicular

- Surgery: thyroid lobectomy or total thyroidectomy if metastases are present.
- Adjunctive treatment: radioactive iodine (^{131}I) for distant metastases and L-thyroxine for replacement therapy to suppress TSH.
- Prognosis: no metastases—90% 10-year survival; metastases—30% 10-year survival.

Anaplastic

- Surgery: only to relieve pressure symptoms.
- Adjunctive treatment: neither radiotherapy nor chemotherapy is effective.
- Prognosis: dismal—most patients will be dead within 12 months of diagnosis.

Medullary

- Exclude phaeochromocytoma before treating.
- Surgery: total thyroidectomy and excision of regional lymph nodes.
- Prognosis: overall 50% 5-year survival.

Aetiology

The following are predisposing factors:

- pre-existing goitre;
- radiation of the neck in childhood.

Clinical features

- Papillary: solitary thyroid nodule.
- Follicular: slow-growing thyroid mass, symptoms from distant metastases.
- Anaplastic: rapidly growing thyroid mass causing tracheal and oesophageal compression.
- Medullary: thyroid lump, may have MEN IIA (medullary thyroid carcinoma, phaeochromocytoma, hyperparathyroidism) or MEN IIB (medullary thyroid carcinoma, phaeochromocytoma, multiple mucosal neuromas, Marfanoid habitus) syndrome.

Investigations

- Ultrasound of the thyroid gland.
- FNAC: may give histological diagnosis.
- Bone scan and radiographs of bones for secondary deposits.
- Calcitonin levels as a marker for medullary carcinoma.

2 Week wait referral criteria for suspected head & neck cancer

- Horseness > 6 weeks
- Oral ulceration > 3 weeks
- Oral swellings > 3 weeks
- Dysphagia > 3 weeks
- Neck mass > 3 weeks
- Cranial neuropathies
- Rapidly developed thyroid lump

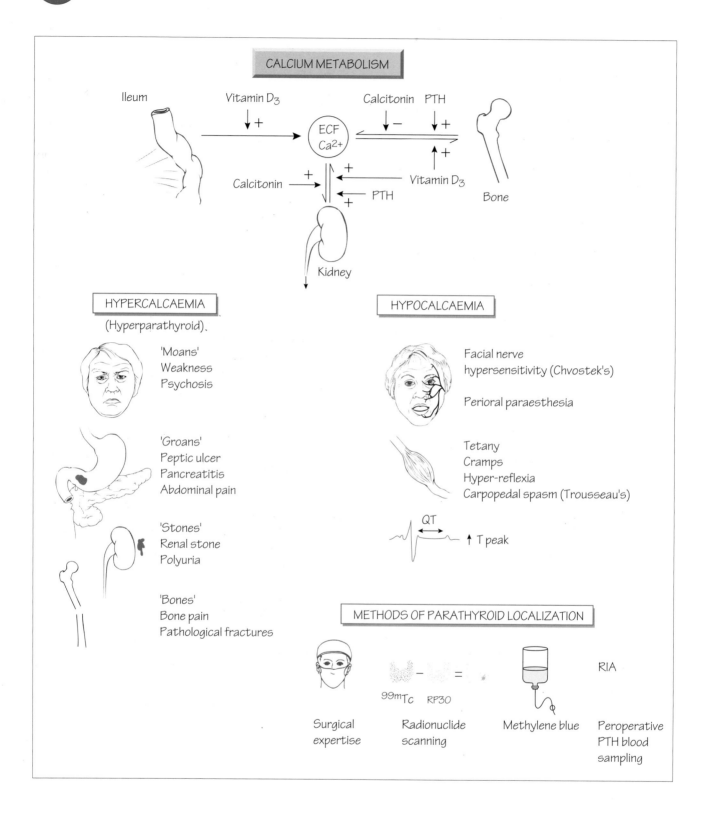

CALCIUM METABOLISM

Ileum — Vitamin D₃ + → ECF Ca²⁺ ← Calcitonin − / PTH + → Bone

Calcitonin + / + PTH / Vitamin D₃ +

Kidney

HYPERCALCAEMIA
(Hyperparathyroid).

'Moans'
Weakness
Psychosis

'Groans'
Peptic ulcer
Pancreatitis
Abdominal pain

'Stones'
Renal stone
Polyuria

'Bones'
Bone pain
Pathological fractures

HYPOCALCAEMIA

Facial nerve
hypersensitivity (Chvostek's)

Perioral paraesthesia

Tetany
Cramps
Hyper-reflexia
Carpopedal spasm (Trousseau's)

QT   ↑ T peak

METHODS OF PARATHYROID LOCALIZATION

⁹⁹ᵐTc   RP30   RIA

Surgical   Radionuclide   Methylene blue   Peroperative
expertise   scanning   PTH blood
                                                      sampling

Hyperparathyroidism

Definition

Hyperparathyroidism is a condition characterized by hypercalcaemia caused by excess production of parathyroid hormone.

Key points

- Hyperparathyroidism often presents with vague symptoms to many different specialists.
- Surgery is the treatment of choice for primary hyperparathyroidism.
- Hypoparathyroidism postsurgery is rare and mostly transient.

Causes

- *Primary* hyperparathyroidism is usually due to a parathyroid adenoma (75%) or parathyroid hyperplasia (20%).
- *Secondary* hyperparathyroidism is hyperplasia of the gland in response to hypocalcaemia (e.g. in chronic renal failure).
- In *tertiary* hyperparathyroidism, autonomous secretion of parathormone occurs when the secondary stimulus has been removed (e.g. after renal transplantation).
- *MEN syndromes* and *ectopic* parathormone production (e.g. oat cell carcinoma of the lung).

Pathology

Parathormone mobilizes calcium from bone, enhances renal tubular absorption and, with vitamin D, intestinal absorption of calcium. The net result is *hypercalcaemia*.

Clinical features

- Renal calculi or renal calcification, polyuria.
- Bone pain, bone deformity, osteitis fibrosa cystica, pathological fractures.
- Muscle weakness, anorexia, intestinal atony, psychosis.
- Peptic ulceration and pancreatitis.

Diagnosis

- Serum calcium (specimen taken on three occasions with patient fasting, at rest and without a tourniquet). Normal range 2.2–2.6 mmol/l. Calcium is bound to albumin and the level has to be 'corrected' when albumin levels are abnormal.
- Parathormone level.
- Imaging:

high-resolution ultrasound;
CT and MRI scanning;
dual isotope imaging (^{201}Tl and ^{99m}Tc pertechnate).
- Selective vein catheterization and digital subtraction angiography in patients in whom exploration has been unsuccessful.

Essential management

- Primary and tertiary hyperparathyroidism are treated surgically: excise adenoma if present, remove $3^{1}/_{2}$ of 4 glands for hyperplasia.
- Secondary hyperplasia: vitamin D and/or calcium.

Hypoparathyroidism

Definition

Hypoparathyroidism is a rare condition characterized by hypocalcaemia due to reduced production of parathormone.

Causes

- Post-thyroid or parathyroid surgery.
- Idiopathic (often autoimmune).
- Congenital enzymatic deficiencies.
- Pseudohypoparathyroidism (reduced sensitivity to parathormone).

Pathology

Reduced serum calcium increases neuromuscular excitability.

Clinical features

- Perioral paraesthesia, cramps, tetany.
- *Chvostek's sign*: tapping over facial nerve induces facial muscle contractions.
- *Trousseau's sign*: inflating BP-cuff to above systolic pressure induces typical *main d'accoucheur* carpal spasm.
- Prolonged QT interval on ECG.

Diagnosis

- Calcium and parathormone levels decreased.

Essential management

Calcium and vitamin D.

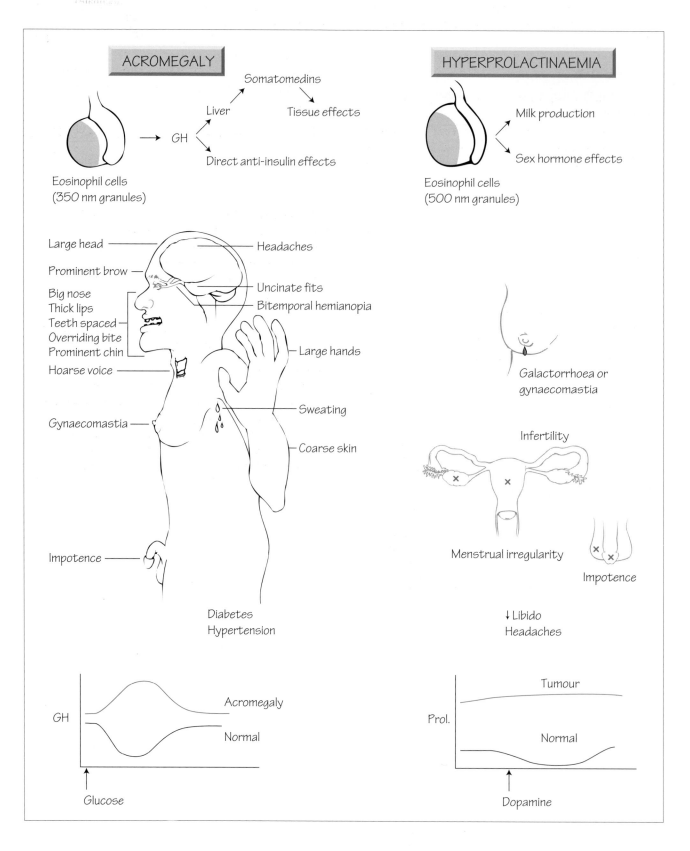

ACROMEGALY

Liver → Somatomedins → Tissue effects

GH → Direct anti-insulin effects

Eosinophil cells
(350 nm granules)

- Large head
- Prominent brow
- Big nose
- Thick lips
- Teeth spaced
- Overriding bite
- Prominent chin
- Hoarse voice
- Gynaecomastia
- Impotence

- Headaches
- Uncinate fits
- Bitemporal hemianopia
- Large hands
- Sweating
- Coarse skin

Diabetes
Hypertension

GH — Acromegaly / Normal

Glucose

HYPERPROLACTINAEMIA

Milk production

Sex hormone effects

Eosinophil cells
(500 nm granules)

Galactorrhoea or
gynaecomastia

Infertility

Menstrual irregularity

Impotence

↓ Libido
Headaches

Prol. — Tumour / Normal

Dopamine

Definition

Pituitary disorders are characterized either by a *failure of secretion* of pituitary hormones or by tumours, which cause local pressure effects or specific syndromes due to hormone overproduction.

Key points

- Acromegaly is often insidious in onset and slow to be diagnosed.
- Deficiencies of pituitary function are generally tested for by stimulation tests and overactivity by suppressions tests. Occasionally direct serum hormone levels may be measured.

Common causes

- Failure of anterior pituitary secretion, pan-hypopituitarism (Simmonds' disease):

  pressure from a tumour;

  infection;

  ischaemia;

  postpartum-induced infarction of the anterior pituitary (Sheehan's syndrome).

Failure of antidiuretic hormone production from the posterior pituitary gland leads to diabetes insipidus:

- trauma;
- local haemorrhage;
- ischaemia;
- tumours.

Tumours (% of total)	Cell type
Endocrinologically active (75%)	
Prolactinomas (35%)	Acidophil
GH-secreting tumours (20%)	Acidophil
Mixed PL and GH (10%)	Acidophil
ACTH-secreting tumours (10%)	Basophil
Endocrinologically inactive (25%)	Chromophobe
Craniopharyngioma	Rathke's pouch

Clinical features

- Pan-hypopituitarism: pallor (MSH), hypothyroid (TSH), failure of lactation (PL), chronic adrenal insufficiency (ACTH), ovarian failure and amenorrhoea (FSH, LH).
- Diabetes insipidus (ADH): polyuria (5–20 l/day), polydipsia.
- Tumours: pressure effects: headache, bitemporal hemianopia.

  Acromegaly (excess GH): thickened skin, increased skull size, prognathism, enlarged tongue, goitre, osteoporosis, organomegaly, spade-like hands and feet.

  Cushing's disease (excess ACTH): malaise, muscle weakness, weight gain, bruising, moon facies, buffalo hump, hirsutism, amenorrhoea, impotence, polyuria, diabetes, emotional instability.

Investigations

- Pan-hypopituitarism: serum assay of pituitary and target gland hormones, dynamic tests of pituitary function.
- Diabetes insipidus: very low urinary specific gravity which does not increase with water deprivation.
- Tumours: visual field measurements, hormone assay, CT or MRI scanning.

Essential management

- Pan-hypopituitarism: replacement therapy—cyclical oestrogen—progesterone, hydrocortisone, thyroxine.
- Diabetes insipidus: vasopressin analogue, desmopressin, administered as nasal spray.
- Tumours: bromocriptine suppresses PL release from prolactinomas, ^{90}Y implant for pituitary ablation, surgery (hypophysectomy via nasal or transcranial route).

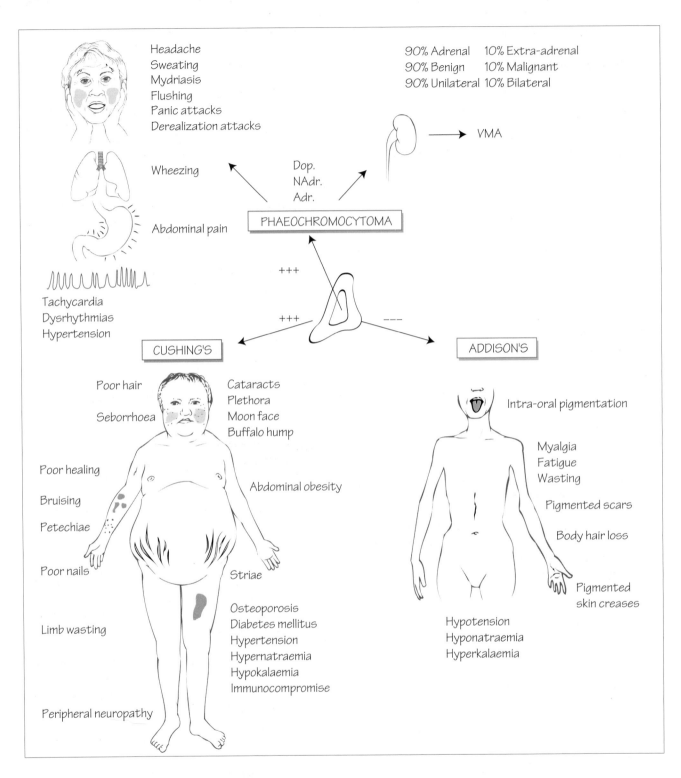

Headache
Sweating
Mydriasis
Flushing
Panic attacks
Derealization attacks

90% Adrenal   10% Extra-adrenal
90% Benign   10% Malignant
90% Unilateral 10% Bilateral

VMA

Wheezing

Dop.
NAdr.
Adr.

Abdominal pain

PHAEOCHROMOCYTOMA

Tachycardia
Dysrhythmias
Hypertension

+++

+++   ---

CUSHING'S   ADDISON'S

Poor hair   Cataracts
                   Plethora
Seborrhoea   Moon face
                   Buffalo hump

Intra-oral pigmentation

Myalgia
Fatigue
Wasting

Poor healing

Bruising

Petechiae

Abdominal obesity

Pigmented scars

Body hair loss

Poor nails   Striae

Osteoporosis
Diabetes mellitus
Hypertension
Hypernatraemia
Hypokalaemia
Immunocompromise

Pigmented
skin creases

Limb wasting

Hypotension
Hyponatraemia
Hyperkalaemia

Peripheral neuropathy

Definitions

Adrenal gland disorders are characterized by clinical syndromes resulting from either a *failure of secretion* or *excessive secretion* of adrenal cortical or medullary hormones.

Cushing's syndrome describes the clinical features irrespective of the cause; *Cushing's disease* refers to a pituitary adenoma with secondary adrenal hyperplasia.

Key points

- Addison's disease is often insidious in onset and presents with vague symptoms—consider in unexplained lethargy and weakness.
- Phaeochromocytoma can mimic a wide range of acute surgical, medical and psychiatric states.
- Cushing's syndrome is commonly caused by chronic exogenous steroid administration.
- Treatment for most situations aims to normalize body physiology before any definitive/surgical treatment is considered.

Common causes

Failure of secretion

Adrenal insufficiency, Addison's disease: bilateral adrenal haemorrhage in sepsis (Waterhouse–Friderichsen syndrome), autoimmune disease, TB, pituitary insufficiency, metastatic deposits.

Excessive secretion

- Cushing's syndrome: excess corticosteroid due to steroid therapy, ACTH-producing pituitary tumour, adenoma or carcinoma of the adrenal cortex, ectopic ACTH production, e.g. oat-cell carcinoma of lung.
- Conn's syndrome (primary hyperaldosteronism): excess aldosterone due to adenoma or carcinoma of adrenal cortex, bilateral cortical hyperplasia.
- Adrenogenital syndrome: excess androgen: abnormal cortisol synthesis causes excess ACTH production which boosts androgen production, adrenal cortical tumour.
- Phaeochromocytoma: excess catecholamines due to adrenal medullary tumours, 95% are benign.

Clinical features

- Addison's disease: see opposite. Addisonian crisis: an acute collapse which may mimic an abdominal emergency.
- Cushing's syndrome: see opposite.
- Conn's syndrome, primary hyperaldosteronism: muscle weakness, tetany, polyuria, polydipsia, hypertension.
- Adrenogenital syndrome: virilization in female children, pseudohermaphroditism, precocious puberty.
- Phaeochromocytoma: see opposite.

Investigations

Basic principles

- Establish the 'endocrine' diagnosis by serum levels or suppressions/stimulation tests.
- Correct the endocrine abnormalities.
- Localize the cause by investigation and imaging.
- Consider if definitive (surgical) treatment is necessary.

Addison's disease

U+Es ($\downarrow$Na$^+$, $\uparrow$K$^+$), low plasma cortisol, short synacthen test to confirm diagnosis. Long synacthen test to differentiate primary (adrenal) from secondary (pituitary) insufficiency.

Cushing's syndrome

Elevated plasma cortisol (taken at 24.00 hours) and loss of diurnal variation, low-dose dexamethasone suppression test to confirm diagnosis, high-dose test to distinguish adrenal from pituitary disease, serum ACTH to identify secondary cause.

Conn's syndrome

U+Es ($\downarrow$K$^+$, normal or $\uparrow$Na$^+$), raised serum aldosterone and normal renin levels.

Adrenogenital syndrome

Elevated urinary 17 ketosteroids.

Phaeochromocytoma

24-hour urinary VMA, serum dopamine, epinephrine (adrenaline) and norepinephrine (noradrenaline).

Localization imaging

- Helical CT: excellent for adrenal gland, retroperitoneum.
- [^{123}I] MIBG scan: neuroendocrine tumours (phaeochromocytoma).
- Arteriography and venous sampling: occasionally required.

Essential management

- Addison's disease: replacement therapy. Cortisol, fludrocortisone. Increase dose at times of stress/surgery.
- Cushing's syndrome: adrenalectomy for adenoma (rarely carcinoma). Mitotane reduces steroid production in metastases.
- Conn's syndrome: adrenalectomy for unilateral adenoma (rarely carcinoma). Spironolactone or amiloride for bilateral adenomas or hyperplasia. (Only if poor response, bilateral adrenalectomy with replacement therapy.)
- Adrenogenital syndrome: cortisol to suppress ACTH and provide corticosteroids. Surgery to correct abnormalities of external genitalia.
- Phaeochromocytoma: surgery after fluid replacement and careful α and β adrenergic blockade.

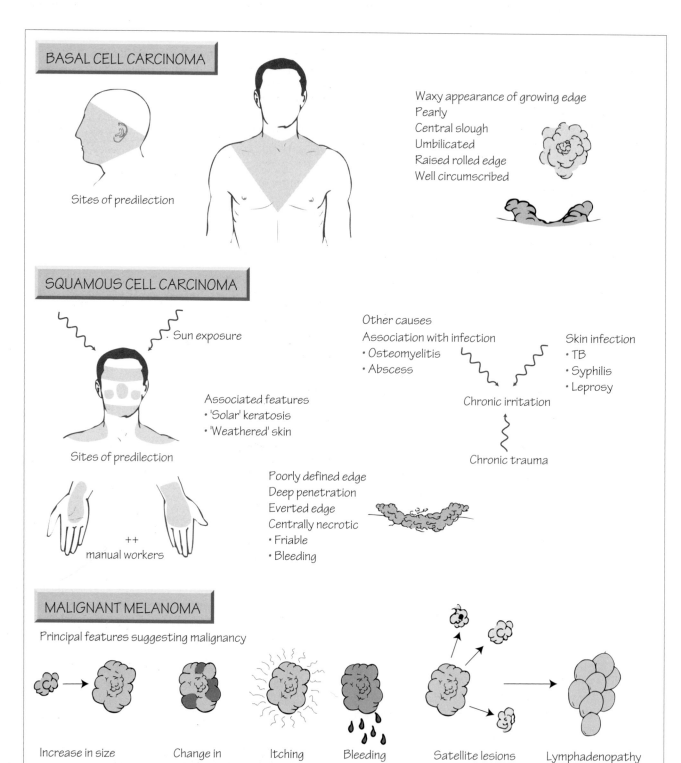

BASAL CELL CARCINOMA

Sites of predilection

Waxy appearance of growing edge
Pearly
Central slough
Umbilicated
Raised rolled edge
Well circumscribed

SQUAMOUS CELL CARCINOMA

Sun exposure

Associated features
• 'Solar' keratosis
• 'Weathered' skin

Sites of predilection

++
manual workers

Other causes
Association with infection
• Osteomyelitis
• Abscess

Skin infection
• TB
• Syphilis
• Leprosy

Chronic irritation

Chronic trauma

Poorly defined edge
Deep penetration
Everted edge
Centrally necrotic
• Friable
• Bleeding

MALIGNANT MELANOMA

Principal features suggesting malignancy

Increase in size

Change in pigmentation

Itching

Bleeding

Satellite lesions

Lymphadenopathy

Definition

Malignant lesions of epidermis of the skin—principally basal cell (BCC) and squamous cell (SCC) carcinomas and malignant melanoma (MM).

Key points

- Protection from sun exposure reduces the risk of all forms of skin cancer dramatically.
- Not all MMs are pigmented.
- All 'moles' with suspicious features should be excision biopsied.
- The prognosis from early MM is excellent with surgery but late disease is usually fatal.

Epidemiology

Male/female 2 : 1 for BCC and SCC. Elderly males. Equal sex distribution and all adults for MM. All tumours common in areas of high annual sunshine (e.g. Australia, southern USA).

Aetiology

The following are predisposing factors.
- Exposure to sunlight (especially in fair-skinned races).
- Immunosuppression (high incidence after renal transplant).
- Radiation exposure (radiotherapy, among radiologists).
- Chemical carcinogens (hydrocarbons, arsenic, coal tar).
- Inherited disorders (albinism, xeroderma pigmentosum).
- Chronic irritation (Marjolin's ulcer).
- Naevi (50% of MM arise in pre-existing benign pigmented lesions).
- Bowen's disease and erythroplasia of Queyrat.

Pathology

BCC
- Arises from basal cells of epidermis.
- Aggressive local spread but do not metastasize.

SCC
- Arises from keratinocytes in the epidermis.
- Spreads by local invasion and metastases.

MM
- Arises from the melanocytes often in pre-existing naevi.
- Superficial spreading and nodular types.
- Radial and vertical growth phases. Lymphatic spread is to regional lymph nodes and haematogenous spread to liver, bone and brain.

Staging

Clarke's levels I–V, Breslow's tumour thickness.

Clinical features

BCC
Recurring, ulcerated, umbilicated skin lesion on forehead or face. Ulcer has a raised, pearl-coloured edge. Untreated, large areas of the face may be eroded (rodent ulcer).

SCC
Lesions (ulcers, fungating lesions with heaped-up edges) on exposed areas of the body.

MM
Pigmented lesions (occasionally not pigmented—amelanotic), 1 cm in diameter on lower limbs, feet, head and neck. Usually present as a change in a pigmented lesion: increasing size or pigmentation/bleeding/pain or itching/ulceration/satellite lesions.

Investigations

- Biopsy (usually excisional) of the lesion unless clinically certain (definitive surgery).
- For MM—helical CT scan for ?involved draining nodes, FNAC for palpable draining nodes, ?peroperative sentinel node biopsy using dye injection mapping.

Essential management

BCC
- Curettage/cautery/cryotherapy/topical chemotherapy (5-FU). These treatments are suitable for small lesions.
- Surgical excision/radiotherapy.

SCC
Surgical excision/radiotherapy.

MM
- Surgical excision with 2–3 cm margin.
- Lymph node dissection if CT, FNAC or sentinel node biopsy +ve for metastases with no systemic disease.
- Immunotherapy, chemotherapy (systemic and local limb perfusion), radiotherapy disseminated disease (poor response).

Prognosis

- BCC, SCC prognosis is usually excellent, but patients with SCC should be followed for 5 years.
- MM prognosis depends on staging:

Clarke's level	5-year survival (%)	Tumour thickness (mm)	5-year survival (%)
I (epidermis)	100	< 0.76	98
II (papillary dermis)	90–100	0.76–1.49	95
III (papillary/ reticular dermis)	80–90	1.50–2.49	80
IV (reticular dermis)	60–70	2.50–3.99	75
V (subcutaneous fat)	15–30	4.00–7.99	60
		> 8.00	40

2 Week wait referral criteria for suspected skin cancer

- Pigmented lesion + increased size/changed shape/changed colour/mixed colour/irregular/ulceration
- Non—healing skin lesion
- Biopsy proven sqamous ca
- New skin lesion in immunosuppressed

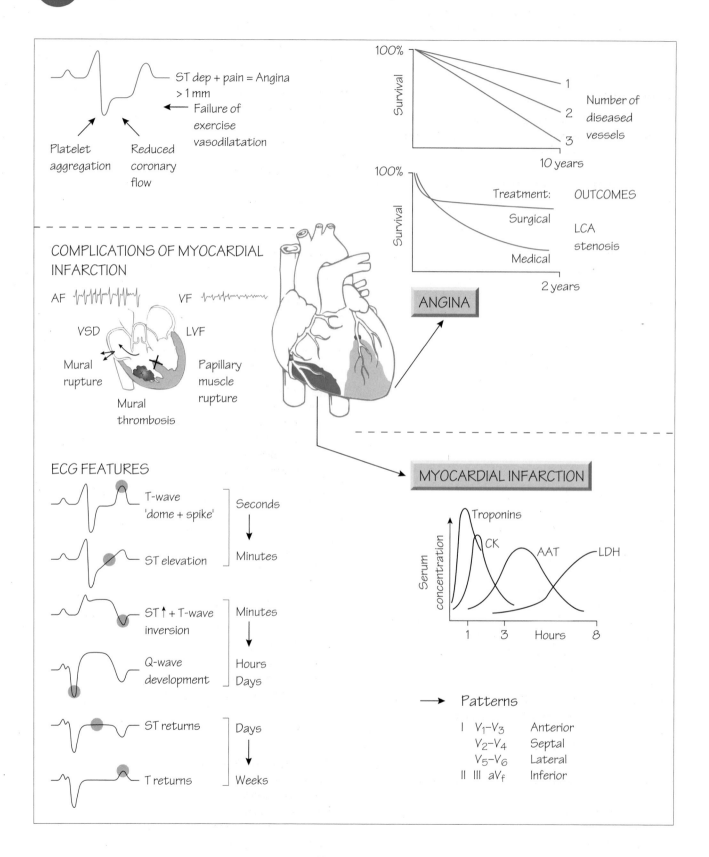

ST dep + pain = Angina
> 1 mm

← Failure of exercise vasodilatation

Platelet aggregation

Reduced coronary flow

Survival
100%
1
2
3
Number of diseased vessels
10 years

Survival
100%
Treatment:
Surgical
Medical
OUTCOMES
LCA stenosis
2 years

ANGINA

COMPLICATIONS OF MYOCARDIAL INFARCTION

AF

VF

VSD

LVF

Mural rupture

Mural thrombosis

Papillary muscle rupture

ECG FEATURES

T-wave 'dome + spike' — Seconds

ST elevation — Minutes

ST↑ + T-wave inversion — Minutes

Q-wave development — Hours / Days

ST returns — Days

T returns — Weeks

MYOCARDIAL INFARCTION

Troponins
CK
AAT
LDH
Serum concentration
1   3   Hours   8

→ Patterns

I	V_1–V_3	Anterior
	V_2–V_4	Septal
	V_5–V_6	Lateral
II III aV_f		Inferior

Definition

Ischaemic heart disease is a common disorder caused by acute or chronic interruption of the blood supply to the myocardium, usually due to atherosclerosis of the coronary arteries, i.e. *coronary artery disease*.

Key points

- Angina alone is rarely managed surgically (CABG).
- Urgent treatment with thrombolysis, antiplatelet agents and cardioprotection reduces the risk of death from MI significantly.
- Serum troponins are highly sensitive and very specific for myocardial injury.

Epidemiology

Male > female before 65 years. Increasing risk with increasing age up to 80 years. Most common cause of death in the Western world.

Aetiology

- Atherosclerosis and thrombosis.
- Thromboemboli (especially plaque rupture).
- Arteritis (e.g. periarteritis nodosa).
- Coronary artery spasm.
- Extension of aortic dissection/syphilitic aortitis.

Risk factors

- Family history.
- Cigarette smoking.
- Hypertension.
- Hyperlipidaemia.
- 'Type A' personality.
- Obesity.

Pathology

- Reduction in coronary blood flow is critical when lumen is decreased by 90%.
- Angina pectoris results when the supply of O_2 to the heart muscle is unable to meet the increased demands for O_2, e.g. during exercise, cold, after a meal.
- Thrombotic occlusion of the narrowed lumen precipitates acute ischaemia.
- The heart muscle in the territory of the occluded vessel dies, i.e. MI. May be subendocardial or transmural.

Clinical features

Angina pectoris

- Central chest pain on exertion, especially in cold weather, lasts 1–15 min.
- Radiates to neck, jaw, arms.
- Relieved by GTN.
- Usually no signs.

Myocardial infarction

- Severe central chest pain for > 30 min duration.
- Radiates to neck, jaw, arms.
- Not relieved by GTN.
- Signs of cardiogenic shock.
- Arrhythmias.

Investigations

Angina pectoris

- FBC: anaemia.
- Thyroid function tests.
- Chest X-ray: heart size.
- ECG ST segment changes.
- Exercise ECG.
- Coronary angiography.

Myocardial infarction

- ECG: Q waves, ST segment and T-wave changes.
- Cardiac enzymes: troponins, LDH, CPK (MB).
- Chest X-ray: dissection.
- FBC: associated anaemia.
- U+E: kyperkalaemia.

Essential management

Angina pectoris

- Lose weight.
- Avoid precipitating factors (e.g. cold).
- GTN (sublingual).
- Calcium channel blockers.
- β-blockers, nitrates, aspirin.
- Treatment of hypertension and hyperlipidaemias.
- Coronary angioplasty or CABG.

Myocardial infarction

- Bed rest, O_2, analgesia.
- Thrombolysis.
- Aspirin.
- Treatment of heart failure.
- Treatment of arrhythmias.

Indications for CABG

- Left main stem disease.
- Triple vessel disease.
- Two-vessel disease involving LAD.
- Chronic ischaemia + LV dysfunction.

Complications of MI

- Arrhythmias.
- Cardiogenic shock.
- Myocardial rupture.
- Papillary muscle rupture causing mitral incompetence.
- Ventricular aneurysm.
- Pericarditis.
- Mural thrombosis and peripheral embolism.

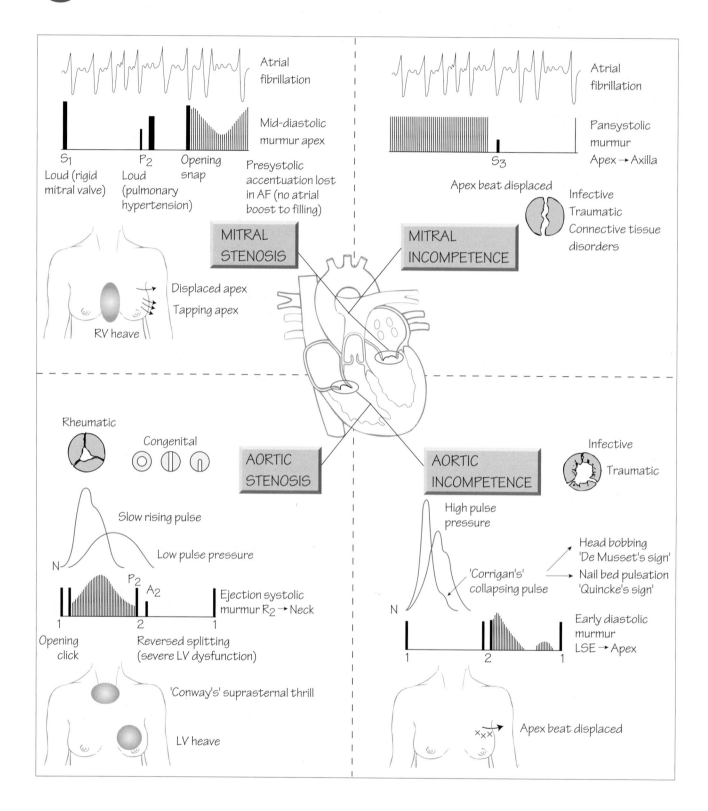

MITRAL STENOSIS

Atrial fibrillation

Mid-diastolic murmur apex

S₁ Loud (rigid mitral valve)
P₂ Loud (pulmonary hypertension)
Opening snap

Presystolic accentuation lost in AF (no atrial boost to filling)

Displaced apex
Tapping apex
RV heave

MITRAL INCOMPETENCE

Atrial fibrillation

Pansystolic murmur Apex → Axilla

S₃

Apex beat displaced

Infective
Traumatic
Connective tissue disorders

AORTIC STENOSIS

Rheumatic
Congenital

Slow rising pulse
Low pulse pressure

P₂ A₂
1 2 1
Ejection systolic murmur R₂ → Neck

Opening click
Reversed splitting (severe LV dysfunction)

'Conway's' suprasternal thrill
LV heave

AORTIC INCOMPETENCE

Infective
Traumatic

High pulse pressure

'Corrigan's' collapsing pulse

Head bobbing 'De Musset's sign'
Nail bed pulsation 'Quincke's sign'

N
1 2 1
Early diastolic murmur LSE → Apex

Apex beat displaced

Definition

Valvular heart disease is defined as a group of conditions characterized by damage to one or more of the heart valves, resulting in deranged blood flow through the heart chambers.

Key point

- Valve replacements are uncommon but offer excellent long-term function with newer bioprosthetic valves.

Epidemiology

Rheumatic fever is still a major problem in developing countries, while congenital heart disease occurs in 8–10 cases per 1000 live births worldwide.

Aetiology

- Congenital valve abnormalities.
- Rheumatic fever.
- Infective endocarditis.
- Degenerative valve disease.

Pathology

- Rheumatic fever—*immune-mediated acute inflammation* affecting the heart valves due to a cross-reaction between antigens of group A α-haemolytic *Streptococcus* and cardiac proteins.
- Disease may make the valve orifice smaller (*stenosis*) or unable to close properly (*incompetence* or *regurgitation*) or both.
- Stenosis causes a *pressure load* while regurgitation causes a *volume load* on the heart chamber immediately proximal to it with upstream and downstream effects.

Clinical features

Aortic stenosis

- Angina pectoris.
- Syncope.
- Left heart failure.
- Slow upstroke arterial pulse.
- Precordial systolic thrill (second right ICS).
- Harsh midsystolic ejection murmur (second right ICS).

Aortic regurgitation

- Congestive cardiac failure.
- Increased pulse pressure.
- Water-hammer pulse.
- Decrescendo diastolic murmur (lower left sternal edge).

Mitral stenosis

- Pulmonary hypertension.
- Paroxysmal nocturnal dyspnoea.
- Atrial fibrillation.
- Loud first heart sound and opening snap.
- Low-pitched diastolic murmur with presystolic accentuation at the apex.

Mitral regurgitation

- Chronic fatigue.
- Pulmonary oedema.
- Apex laterally displaced, hyperdynamic praecordium.
- Apical pansystolic murmur radiating to axilla.

Tricuspid stenosis

- Fatigue.
- Peripheral oedema.
- Liver enlargement/ascites.
- Prominent JVP with large a waves.
- Lung fields are clear.
- Rumbling diastolic murmur (lower left sternal border).

Tricuspid regurgitation

- Chronic fatigue.
- Hepatomegaly/ascites.
- Right ventricular heave.
- Prominent JVP with large v waves.
- Pansystolic murmur (subxiphoid area).

Investigations

- ECG.
- Chest X-ray.
- Echocardiography and colour Doppler techniques.
- Cardiac catheterization with measurement of transvalvular gradients.

Essential managemenet

Medical

Treat cardiac failure, diuretics, restrict salt intake, reduce exercise, digitalis for rapid atrial fibrillation and anticoagulation for peripheral embolization.

Surgical

Repair (possible in mitral and tricuspid valve only) or replace diseased valve (requires cardiopulmonary bypass). *Prosthetic* (lifelong anticoagulation), *bioprosthetic* (animal tissue on prosthetic frame, 3 months' anticoagulation) and *biological* (cadaveric homografts, no anticoagulation) valves available.

CHRONIC ISCHAEMIA

AORTO-ILIAC FEMORO-POPLITEAL INFRA-POPLITEAL

Sites affected

Buttocks
Thighs
Pelvis
(including sex organs)

Thighs
Calves

Calves
Feet

Pulses affected

Treatment options

Balloon angioplasty

Balloon angioplasty

Saphenous vein
in situ or reversed
5-year patency
<60%

Intraluminal stent

Only for profunda
origin disease

Endarterectomy + profundaplasty

Femoro-distal vein graft

5-year patency 90%

Saphenous vein
in situ or reversed
5-year patency 70–80%

Femoro-popliteal vein graft

Anatomical grafts
• Aorto-bi-iliac
• Aorto-bifemoral

5-year patency 60%

Gortex ± armoured
5-year patency 60–70%

Femoro-popliteal synthetic graft

Extra-anatomical grafts
• Axillo-bifemoral
• Femoro-femoral

Definition

Peripheral occlusive vascular disease (POVD) is a common disorder caused by acute or chronic interruption of the blood supply to the limbs, usually due to atherosclerosis.

Key points

- All patients with POVD require screening for associated coronary or carotid disease.
- The majority of POVD responds to conservative treatment.
- Surgery is confined to limb-threatening (critical) ischaemia or truly disabling, refractory claudication.

Epidemiology

Male > female before 65 years. Increased risk with increased age.

Aetiology

- Atherosclerosis and thrombosis.
- Embolism.
- Vascular trauma.
- Vasculitis (e.g. Buerger's disease).

Risk factors

- Cigarette smoking.
- Hypertension.
- Hyperlipidaemia.
- Diabetes mellitus.
- Family history.

Pathology

Reduction in blood flow to the peripheral tissues results in ischaemia which may be acute or chronic. Critical ischaemia is present when the reduction of blood flow is such that tissue viability cannot be sustained (defined by tissue loss, rest pain for 2 weeks, ankle pressure < 50 mmHg).

Clinical features

Chronic ischaemia (see p. 50)

- Intermittent claudication in calf (femoral), thigh (iliac) or buttock (aortoiliac).
- Cold peripheries.
- Prolonged capillary refill time.
- Rest pain, especially at night.
- Venous guttering.
- Absent pulses.
- Arterial ulcers, especially over pressure points (heels, toes).
- Knee contractures.

Acute ischaemia (see p. 54)

- Pain.
- Pallor.
- Pulselessness.
- Paraesthesia.
- Paralysis.
- 'Perishing' cold.
- 'Pistol shot' onset.
- Mottling.
- Muscle rigidity.

Investigations

Chronic ischaemia

- ABI (normal >1.0) at rest and postexercise on treadmill.
- FBC (exclude polycythaemia).
- Doppler wave-form analysis.
- Digital plethysmography (in diabetes).
- Perfemoral angiography.

Acute ischaemia

- ECG, cardiac enzymes.
- Angiography (?), may be performed peroperatively.
- Find source of embolism. Holter monitoring. Echocardiograph. Ultrasound aorta for AAA.

Essential management

Non-disabling claudication

- Stop smoking.
- Exercise programme.
- Avoid β-blockers.
- Aspirin 75 mg/day.
- Statin.
- Cilostazol 100 mg twice daily—improves claudication distance (contraindicated in patients with CCF).

Disabling claudication/critical ischaemia

- Balloon angioplasty ± intravascular stent.
- Bypass surgery.
- Amputation.
- i.v. treatment: iloprost.

Acute ischaemia

- Heparin anticoagulation.
- Surgical embolectomy.
- Thrombolytic therapy (t-PA, streptokinase, urokinase).

Prognosis

Non-disabling claudication

> 65% respond to conservative management. The rest require more aggressive treatment.

Disabling claudication/critical ischaemia

- Angioplasty and bypass surgery overall give good results.
- The more distal the anastomosis the poorer the result.

Acute ischaemia

- Limb salvage 85%.
- Mortality 10–15%.

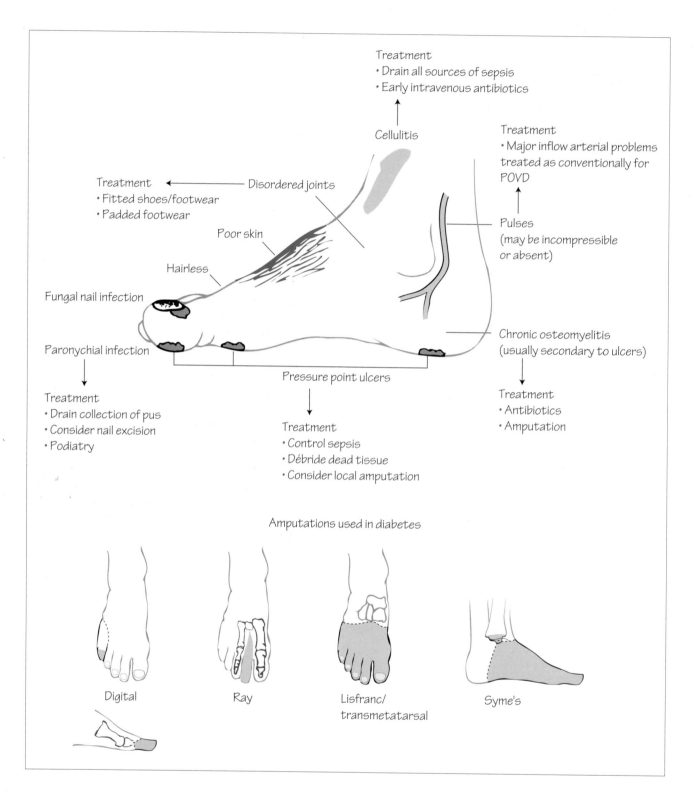

Treatment
• Drain all sources of sepsis
• Early intravenous antibiotics

Cellulitis

Treatment
• Major inflow arterial problems treated as conventionally for POVD

Treatment
• Fitted shoes/footwear
• Padded footwear

Disordered joints

Poor skin

Pulses
(may be incompressible or absent)

Hairless

Fungal nail infection

Paronychial infection

Chronic osteomyelitis
(usually secondary to ulcers)

Pressure point ulcers

Treatment
• Drain collection of pus
• Consider nail excision
• Podiatry

Treatment
• Control sepsis
• Débride dead tissue
• Consider local amputation

Treatment
• Antibiotics
• Amputation

Amputations used in diabetes

Digital

Ray

Lisfranc/
transmetatarsal

Syme's

Definition

The term *diabetic foot* refers to a spectrum of foot disorders ranging from ulceration to gangrene occurring in diabetic people as a result of peripheral neuropathy or ischaemia, or both.

Key points

- Prevention is everything in diabetic feet.
- All infections should be treated aggressively to reduce the risk of tissue loss.
- Treat major vessel POVD as normal—improve 'inflow' to the foot.

Pathophysiology

Three distinct processes lead to the problem of the diabetic foot.
- *Ischaemia* caused by macro- and microangiopathy.
- *Neuropathy*: sensory, motor and autonomic.
- *Sepsis*: the glucose-saturated tissue promotes bacterial growth.

Clinical features

Neuropathic features

- Sensory disturbances.
- Trophic skin changes.
- Plantar ulceration.
- Degenerative arthropathy (Charcot's joints).
- Pulses often present.
- Sepsis (bacterial/fungal).

Ischaemic features

- Rest pain.
- Painful ulcers over pressure areas.
- History of intermittent claudication.
- Absent pulses.
- Sepsis (bacterial/fungal).

Investigations

- Non-invasive vascular tests: ABI, segmental pressure, digital pressure. ABI may be falsely elevated due to medial sclerosis.
- X-ray of foot may show osteomyelitis.
- Arteriography.

Essential management

Should be undertaken jointly by surgeon and physician as diabetic foot may precipitate diabetic ketoacidosis. Diabetic patients should be prescribed an antiplatelet agent and a statin.

Prevention
Do
- Carefully wash and dry feet daily.
- Inspect feet daily.
- Take meticulous care of toenails.
- Use antifungal powder.

Do not
- Walk barefoot.
- Wear ill-fitting shoes.
- Use a hot water bottle.
- Ignore any foot injury.

Neuropathic disease
- Control infection with antibiotics effective against both aerobes and anaerobes.
- Wide local excision and drainage of necrotic tissue.
- These measures usually result in healing.

Ischaemic disease
- Formal assessment of the vascular tree by angiography and reconstitution of the blood supply to the foot (either by angioplasty or bypass surgery) must be achieved before the local measures will work.
- After restoration of blood supply treat as for neuropathic disease.

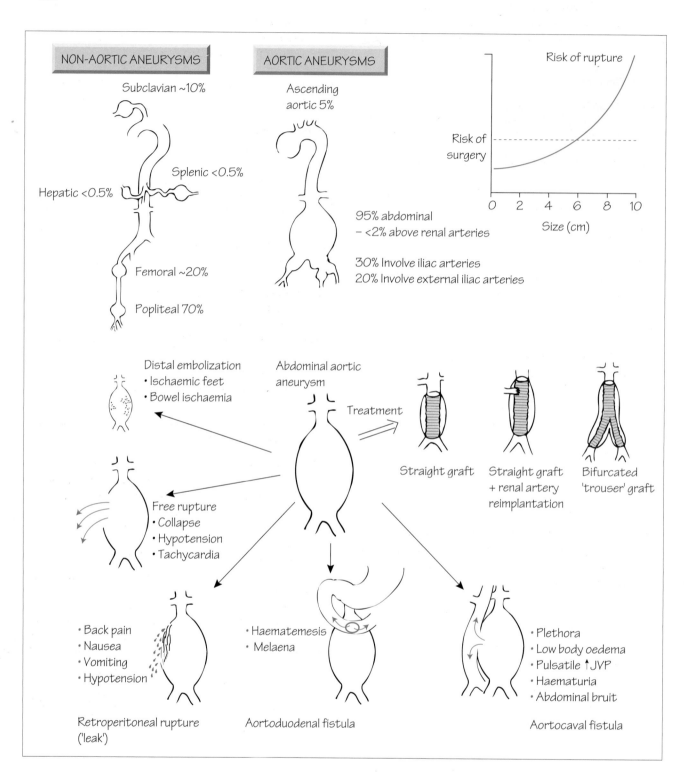

NON-AORTIC ANEURYSMS

Subclavian ~10%

Splenic <0.5%

Hepatic <0.5%

Femoral ~20%

Popliteal 70%

AORTIC ANEURYSMS

Ascending aortic 5%

95% abdominal – <2% above renal arteries

30% Involve iliac arteries
20% Involve external iliac arteries

Risk of rupture

Risk of surgery

Size (cm)

Distal embolization
• Ischaemic feet
• Bowel ischaemia

Abdominal aortic aneurysm

Treatment

Straight graft

Straight graft + renal artery reimplantation

Bifurcated 'trouser' graft

Free rupture
• Collapse
• Hypotension
• Tachycardia

• Back pain
• Nausea
• Vomiting
• Hypotension

Retroperitoneal rupture ('leak')

• Haematemesis
• Melaena

Aortoduodenal fistula

• Plethora
• Low body oedema
• Pulsatile ↑JVP
• Haematuria
• Abdominal bruit

Aortocaval fistula

Definitions

An *aneurysm* is a permanent localized dilatation of an artery to the extent that the affected artery is 1.5 times its normal diameter. A *pseudo* or *false aneurysm* is an expanding pulsating haematoma in continuity with a vessel lumen. It does not have an epithelial lining.

Key points

- All patients with other vascular disease should be examined for AAA.
- Regular monitoring of size helps determine timing for elective surgery.
- Mortality for elective surgery is reduced by careful patient evaluation for hidden coronary or pulmonary disease.

Sites

Abdominal aorta, iliac, femoral and popliteal arteries. Cerebral and thoracic aneurysms are less common.

Aetiology

- Atherosclerosis.
- Familial (abnormal collagenase or elastase activity).
- Congenital (cerebral (berry) aneurysm).
- Bacterial aortitis (mycotic aneurysm).
- Syphilitic aortitis (thoracic aneurysm).

Risk factors

- Cigarette smoking.
- Hypertension.
- Hyperlipidaemia.

Pathology

- Aneurysms increase in size in line with the law of Laplace ($T = RP$), T = tension on the arterial wall, R = radius of artery, P = blood pressure. Increasing tension leads to rupture.
- Thrombus from within an aneurysm may be a source of peripheral emboli.
- Popliteal aneurysms may undergo complete thrombosis leading to acute leg ischaemia.
- Aneurysms may be fusiform (AAA, popliteal) or saccular (thoracic, cerebral).

Clinical features of AAA

Asymptomatic

The vast majority have no symptoms and are found incidentally.

This has led to the description of an AAA as 'a U-boat in the belly'.

Symptomatic

- Back pain from pressure on the vertebral column.
- Rapid expansion causes flank or back pain.
- Rupture causes collapse, back pain and an ill-defined mass.
- Erosion into IVC causes CCF, loud abdominal bruit (machinery murmur), lower limb ischaemia and gross oedema.

Investigations

Detection of AAA

- Physical examination: not accurate.
- Plain abdominal X-ray: aortic calcification.
- Ultrasonography: best way of detecting and measuring aneurysm size.
- CT scan: provides good information regarding relationship between AAA and renal arteries.
- Angiography: not routine for AAA.

Determination of fitness for surgery

- History and examination.
- ECG ± stress testing.
- Radionuclide cardiac scanning (MUGA or stress thallium scan).
- Pulmonary function tests.
- U+E and creatinine for renal assessment.

Essential management

- Surgical repair is the treatment of choice for AAA.
- AAA of ≥ 5.5 cm should be repaired electively as they have a high rate of rupture (perioperative mortality for elective AAA repair is 5%). AAA < 5.5 cm may be monitored with serial ultrasound examinations every 6 months.
- Surgical repair with inlay of a synthetic graft is the standard method of repair.
- Endovascular repair with graft/stent devices is indicated in selected patients.
- Ruptured AAA require immediate surgical repair (perioperative mortality 50%, but 70% of patients die before they get to hospital so that overall mortality is 85%).

Prognosis

Most patients do well after surviving AAA repair and have an excellent quality of life.

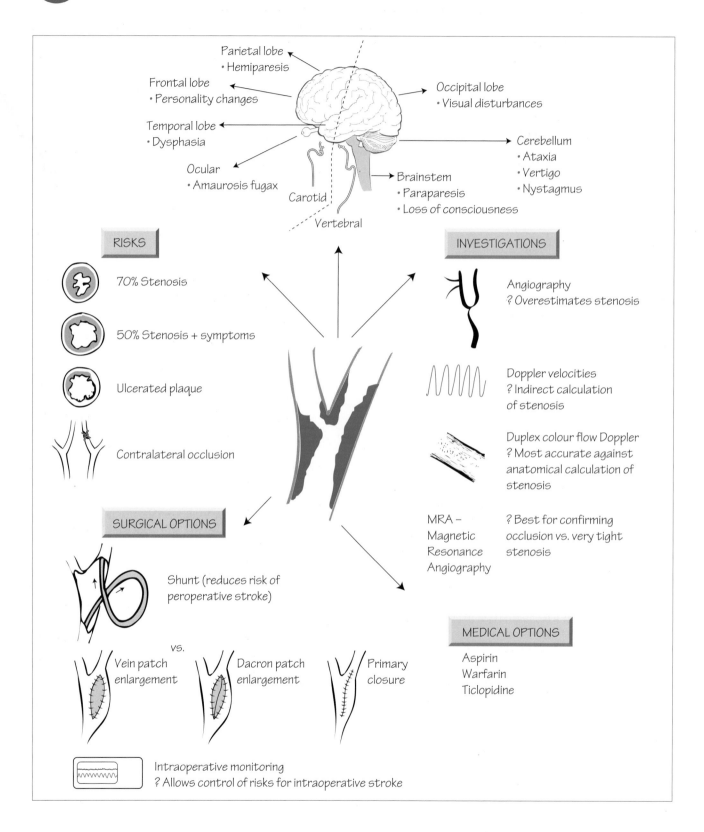

Parietal lobe
• Hemiparesis

Frontal lobe
• Personality changes

Temporal lobe
• Dysphasia

Ocular
• Amaurosis fugax

Carotid

Vertebral

Occipital lobe
• Visual disturbances

Cerebellum
• Ataxia
• Vertigo
• Nystagmus

Brainstem
• Paraparesis
• Loss of consciousness

RISKS

70% Stenosis

50% Stenosis + symptoms

Ulcerated plaque

Contralateral occlusion

INVESTIGATIONS

Angiography
? Overestimates stenosis

Doppler velocities
? Indirect calculation
of stenosis

Duplex colour flow Doppler
? Most accurate against
anatomical calculation of
stenosis

MRA –
Magnetic
Resonance
Angiography

? Best for confirming
occlusion vs. very tight
stenosis

SURGICAL OPTIONS

Shunt (reduces risk of
peroperative stroke)

vs.

Vein patch
enlargement

Dacron patch
enlargement

Primary
closure

MEDICAL OPTIONS

Aspirin
Warfarin
Ticlopidine

Intraoperative monitoring
? Allows control of risks for intraoperative stroke

Definition

Extracranial arterial disease is a common disorder characterized by atherosclerosis of the carotid or vertebral arteries resulting in cerebral-ocular (*stroke, TIA, amaurosis fugax*) or cerebellar (vertigo, ataxia, drop attacks) ischaemic symptoms.

Key points

- All patients with transient neurological symptoms should undergo screening for carotid disease—clinical examination is not accurate.
- Targeted carotid endarterectomy offers optimal risk benefit in stroke prevention.

Epidemiology

Male > female before 65 years. Increasing risk with increasing age.

Aetiology

- Atherosclerosis and thrombosis.
- Thromboemboli.
- Fibromuscular dysplasia.

Risk factors

- Cigarette smoking.
- Hypertension.
- Hyperlipidaemia.

Pathophysiology

- The most common extracranial lesion is an atherosclerotic plaque at the carotid bifurcation. Platelet aggregation and subsequent *platelet embolization* cause ocular or cerebral symptoms.
- Symptoms due to *flow reduction* are rare in the carotid territory, but vertebrobasilar symptoms are usually flow related. Reversed flow in the vertebral artery in the presence of ipsilateral subclavian occlusion leads to cerebral symptoms as the arm 'steals' blood from the cerebellum – subclavian steal syndrome.

Clinical features

- Cerebral symptoms (contralateral):
  motor (weakness, clumsiness or paralysis of a limb);
  sensory (numbness, paraesthesia);
  speech related (receptive or expressive dysphasia).
- Ocular symptoms (ipsilateral): amaurosis fugax (transient loss of vision described as a veil coming down over the visual field).
- Cerebral (or ocular) symptoms may be transitory (a *transient ischaemic attack* is a focal neurological or ocular deficit lasting not more than 24 hours) or permanent (a *stroke*).
- Vertebrobasilar symptoms: vertigo, ataxia, dizziness, syncope, bilateral paraesthesia, visual hallucinations.
- A *bruit* may be heard over a carotid artery, but it is an unreliable indicator of pathology.

Investigations

- Duplex scanning: B-mode scan and Doppler ultrasonic velocitometry: method of choice for assessing degree of carotid stenosis.
- Carotid angiography: Now often performed as MRA, which is safer than standard angiography. Not essential prior to surgery.
- CT or MRI brain scan: demonstrate the presence of a cerebral infarct.

Essential management

Medical

- Aspirin (75 mg/day) inhibits platelet aggregation for the life of the platelet.
- Clopidogril (75 mg/day) has a similar action to aspirin.
- All patients with evidence of vascular disease should be prescribed a statin.
- Anticoagulation is indicated in patients with cardiac embolic disease.

Surgical

- Carotid endarterectomy (+ aspirin).

Indications for carotid endarterectomy

- Carotid distribution TIA or stroke with good recovery after 1-month delay:
  >70% ipsilateral stenosis;
  >50% ipsilateral stenosis with ulceration.
- Asymptomatic carotid stenosis > 80% (controversial).
- Carotid endarterectomy has about 5% morbidity and mortality.
- Carotid angioplasty ± stenting, using a protection device to prevent distal embolisation during the procedure, is currently being evaluated.

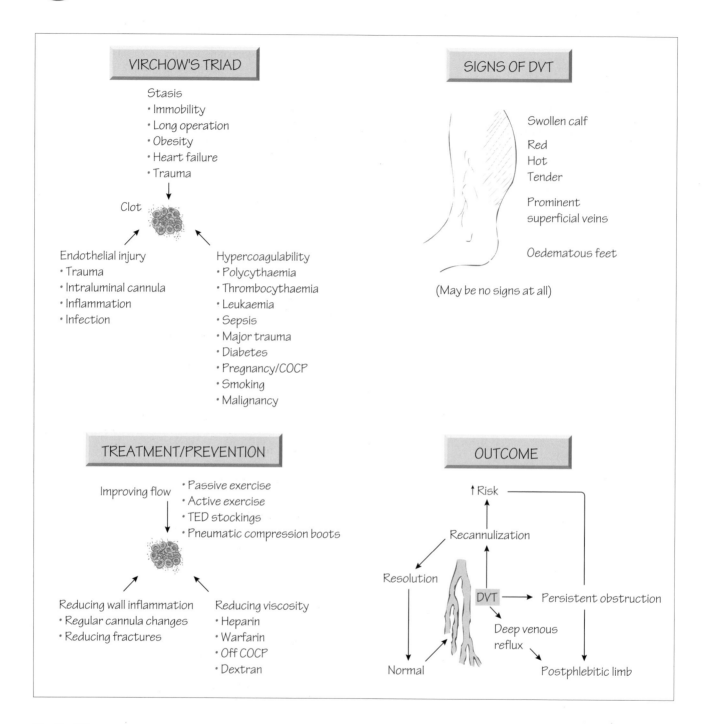

VIRCHOW'S TRIAD

Stasis
• Immobility
• Long operation
• Obesity
• Heart failure
• Trauma

Clot

Endothelial injury
• Trauma
• Intraluminal cannula
• Inflammation
• Infection

Hypercoagulability
• Polycythaemia
• Thrombocythaemia
• Leukaemia
• Sepsis
• Major trauma
• Diabetes
• Pregnancy/COCP
• Smoking
• Malignancy

SIGNS OF DVT

Swollen calf

Red
Hot
Tender

Prominent
superficial veins

Oedematous feet

(May be no signs at all)

TREATMENT/PREVENTION

Improving flow
• Passive exercise
• Active exercise
• TED stockings
• Pneumatic compression boots

Reducing wall inflammation
• Regular cannula changes
• Reducing fractures

Reducing viscosity
• Heparin
• Warfarin
• Off COCP
• Dextran

OUTCOME

↑ Risk
Recannulization
Resolution
DVT → Persistent obstruction
Deep venous reflux
Normal
Postphlebitic limb

Definitions

A *deep venous thrombosis* (DVT) is a condition in which the blood in the deep veins of the legs or pelvis clots. Embolization of the thrombus results in a *pulmonary embolus* (PE) while local venous damage may lead to chronic venous hypertension and the *postphlebitic limb* (PPL).

Key points

• All patients in hospital should be considered for mechanical and pharmacological DVT prophylaxis.
• Have a low threshold of investigation for DVT in bed-bound patients.
• Recurrent DVT may lead to chronic disabling postphlebitic limb.
• DVT may be the first manifestation of an occult malignancy.

Epidemiology

DVT is extremely common among medical and surgical patients, affecting 10–30% of all general surgical patients over 40 years who undergo a major operation. PE is a common cause of sudden death in hospital patients (0.5–3.0% of patients die from PE).

Aetiology
Risk factors
- Increasing age > 40 years.
- Immobilization.
- Obesity.
- Malignancy.
- Sepsis.
- Thrombophilia (e.g. antithrombin III/protein C/protein S deficiency, Factor V leiden, anticardiolipin Ab).
- Inflammatory bowel disease.
- Trauma.
- Heart disease.
- Pregnancy/oestrogens.

Virchow's triad
- Stasis.
- Endothelial injury.
- Hypercoagulability.

Pathology
- Aggregation of platelets in valve pockets (area of maximum stasis or injury).
- Activation of clotting cascade producing fibrin.
- Fibrin production overwhelms the natural anticoagulant/ fibrinolytic system.
- Natural history.
- Complete resolution vs. PE vs. PPL.

Clinical features
DVT
- Asymptomatic.
- Calf tenderness, ankle oedema, mild pyrexia,
- Phlegmasia alba/caerulea dolens.

PE
- Substernal chest pain.
- Dyspnoea.
- Circulatory arrest.
- Pleuritic chest pain.
- Haemoptysis.

PPL
- History of DVT.
- Aching limb.
- Leg swelling.
- Venous eczema.
- Venous ulceration.
- Inverted bottle-shaped leg.

Investigations
DVT
- D-dimers.
- Duplex imaging—suprapopliteal thrombosis.
- Ascending venography.

PE
- ECG: S1, Q3, T3.
- Chest X-ray: linear collapse.
- Blood gases: hypoxia, hypocapnia.
- Ventilation/perfusion lung scan.
- Pulmonary angiography.

PPL
- Ascending ± descending venography.
- Duplex scanning.
- Plethysmography.
- Ambulatory venous pressure.

Essential management

Prophylaxis against DVT
Indications
Presence of risk factors (see above).

Methods
- Mechanical compression (TED) stockings.
- Pharmacological subcutaneous heparin 5000 IU s.c. b.d. (warfarin 1 mg/day, dextran 70 i.v., 500 ml/day).

Definitive treatment
DVT
- Anticoagulation for 6–8 weeks:
  i.v. heparin (check efficacy with APTT);
  warfarin (check efficacy with PT).
- (Thrombolysis.)
- (Thrombectomy.)

PE
- Anticoagulation for 3–6 months.
- Thrombolysis.
- Pulmonary embolectomy.
- IVC filters for recurrent PE despite treatment, anticoagulation treatment contraindicated, 'high risk' DVTs.

PPL
- Limb elevation.
- Compression.
- Four-layer bandaging to achieve ulcer healing.
- Graduated compression stockings to maintain limb compression.
- (Venous valve reconstruction.)

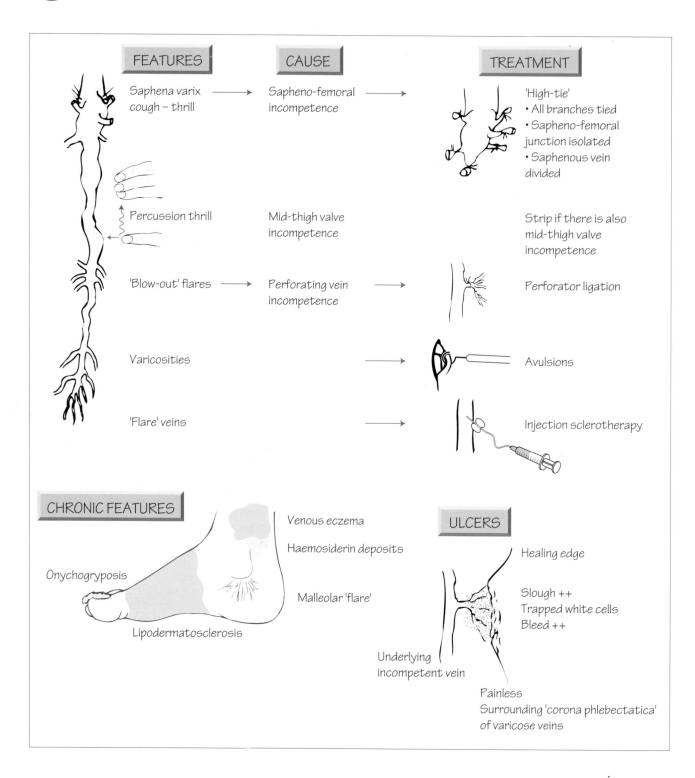

FEATURES

Saphena varix
cough – thrill

Percussion thrill

'Blow-out' flares

Varicosities

'Flare' veins

CAUSE

Sapheno-femoral
incompetence

Mid-thigh valve
incompetence

Perforating vein
incompetence

TREATMENT

'High-tie'
• All branches tied
• Sapheno-femoral
  junction isolated
• Saphenous vein
  divided

Strip if there is also
mid-thigh valve
incompetence

Perforator ligation

Avulsions

Injection sclerotherapy

CHRONIC FEATURES

Venous eczema

Haemosiderin deposits

Malleolar 'flare'

Onychogryposis

Lipodermatosclerosis

ULCERS

Healing edge

Slough ++
Trapped white cells
Bleed ++

Underlying
incompetent vein

Painless
Surrounding 'corona phlebectatica'
of varicose veins

Definition

Varicose veins are tortuous, dilated prominent superficial veins in the lower limbs, often in the anatomical distribution of the long and short saphenous veins.

Key points

- Surgery for varicose veins aims to divide all incompetent perforators and remove grossly diseased varicosities.
- Smaller varicose veins are best treated by injection sclerotherapy alone.
- Beware non-anatomical or atypical varicose veins in the young adult (congenital causes).
- Recurrent varicose veins require Duplex scanning assessment.

Epidemiology

Very common in the Western world, affecting about 50% of the adult population.

Aetiology

- Primary or familial varicose veins.
- Pregnancy (progesterone causes passive dilatation of veins).
- Secondary to postphlebitic limb (perforator failure).
- Congenital:
  Klippel–Trenaunay syndrome;
  Parkes–Weber syndrome.
- Iatrogenic: following formation of an arteriovenous fistula.

Pathophysiology

Venous valve failure, usually at the sapheno-femoral junction (and sometimes in perforating veins), results in increased venous pressure in the long saphenous vein with progressive vein dilatation and further valve disruption.

Clinical features

- Asymptomatic.
- Cosmetic appearance.
- Dull aching leg pain. ⎫ Symptoms worse in the evening
- Heaviness in the leg. ⎭ or on standing for long periods.
- Itching and eczema.
- Superficial thrombophlebitis.
- Bleeding.
- Saphena varix.
- Ulceration.

Investigations

- Clinical assessment by Trendelenburg tourniquet tests.
- Doppler velocitometry: assess sapheno-femoral junction (SFJ)/short sapheno-popliteal junction (SSPJ).
- Duplex scanning: identify recurrence site (especially recurrent varicose veins).

Essential management

General

- Avoid long periods of standing.
- Elevate limbs.
- Wear support hosiery.

Specific

Injection sclerotherapy with sodium tetradecyl (STD)

- Suitable for small veins and usually only below the knee.
- Patients are encouraged to walk several miles per day.
- Anaphylaxis and local ulceration may occur.

Surgical ablation

- With the patient standing, the dilated veins are carefully marked with an indelible marker.
- The saphenous vein is surgically disconnected from the femoral vein and the perforators are also ablated.
- The elongated veins are removed via multiple stab incisions and long segments above the knee are removed using a 'vein stripper'.
- Postoperatively compression stockings are worn for several weeks and exercise is encouraged.
- Surgery is the most effective treatment for large varicose veins, but recurrence rates are high.

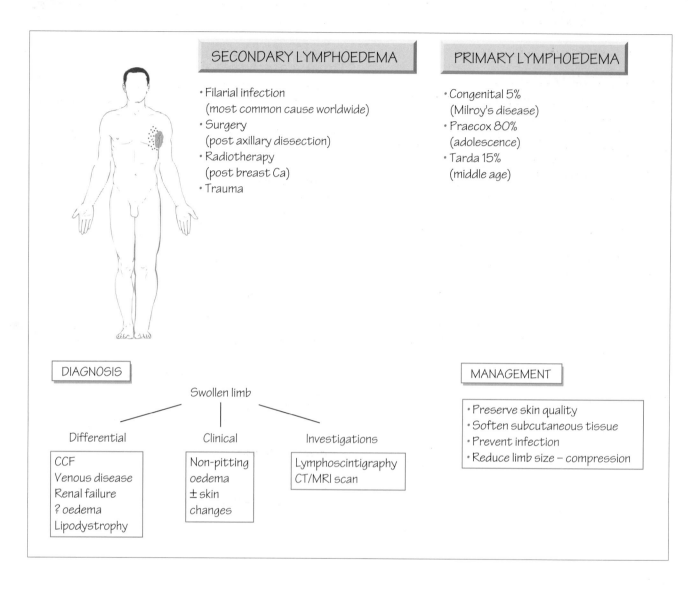

SECONDARY LYMPHOEDEMA

• Filarial infection
  (most common cause worldwide)
• Surgery
  (post axillary dissection)
• Radiotherapy
  (post breast Ca)
• Trauma

PRIMARY LYMPHOEDEMA

• Congenital 5%
  (Milroy's disease)
• Praecox 80%
  (adolescence)
• Tarda 15%
  (middle age)

DIAGNOSIS

Swollen limb

Differential

CCF
Venous disease
Renal failure
? oedema
Lipodystrophy

Clinical

Non-pitting
oedema
± skin
changes

Investigations

Lymphoscintigraphy
CT/MRI scan

MANAGEMENT

• Preserve skin quality
• Soften subcutaneous tissue
• Prevent infection
• Reduce limb size – compression

Definition

Lymphoedema is a persistent swelling of the tissues caused by the accumulation of protein-rich fluid as a result of failure of lymph transport from the tissues.

Classification of lymphoedema

Lymphoedema	Lymphatic defect
Primary (uncommon)	
Congenital (Milroy's disease) (rare)	Aplasia (15%)
Praecox—appears in adolescence (80% of primary lymphoedema)	Hypoplasia (70%)
Tarda—appears in middle age	Hyperplasia/varicosity (15%)
Secondary (common)	
Infection (Filariasis*, TB, lymphogranuloma, actinomycosis. chronic lymphangitis.	Hyperplastic/varicose
Surgery (especially after axillary dissection for breast cancer)	
Radiation therapy (especially for breast cancer)	
Trauma	

TB = tuberculosis *Parasitic infestation with filarial worm *Wuchereria bancrofti.*

Clinical features

Limb swelling

- Starts distally and ascends proximally over period of months.
- Characteristic 'tree trunk' appearance to lower limb.
- Absence of pigmentation differentiates lower limb lymphoedema from venous insufficiency.

Clinical grades

- Grade 1—pitting oedema and decrease in swelling on limb elevation.
- Grade 2—non-pitting oedema and little decrease in swelling on elevation.
- Grade 3—(elephantiasis) gross swelling of the limb with skin changes.

Investigations

- Diagnosis is usually made on history and clinical examination.
- (Lymphangiography)—not used anymore.
- Lymphscintigriphy—best method of measuring lymphatic function.
- CT or MR scanning of limb—good for imaging oedema and fibrosis.

Management

Lymphoedema is a chronic condition that cannot be cured but it can be managed.

Aims of management are to:
- Preserve skin quality.
- Soften subcutaneous tissue.
- Prevent lymphangitis.
- Reduce limb size.

Complex physical therapy:
- Skin care to avoid infection and further lymphatic damage.
- Massage therapy and exercise to promote lymph flow.
- Compression bandages and garments to decrease limb size.
- External pneumatic compression to decrease limb size.

Drug therapy:
- Benzopyrones, flavonoids, antibiotics, diuretics (all have been used but usefulness unproven, benzopyrones may cause hepatic impairment)

Surgery (rarely indicated):
- Liposuction.
- Lymphangiectomy.
- Lymphatico-venous anastomosis.

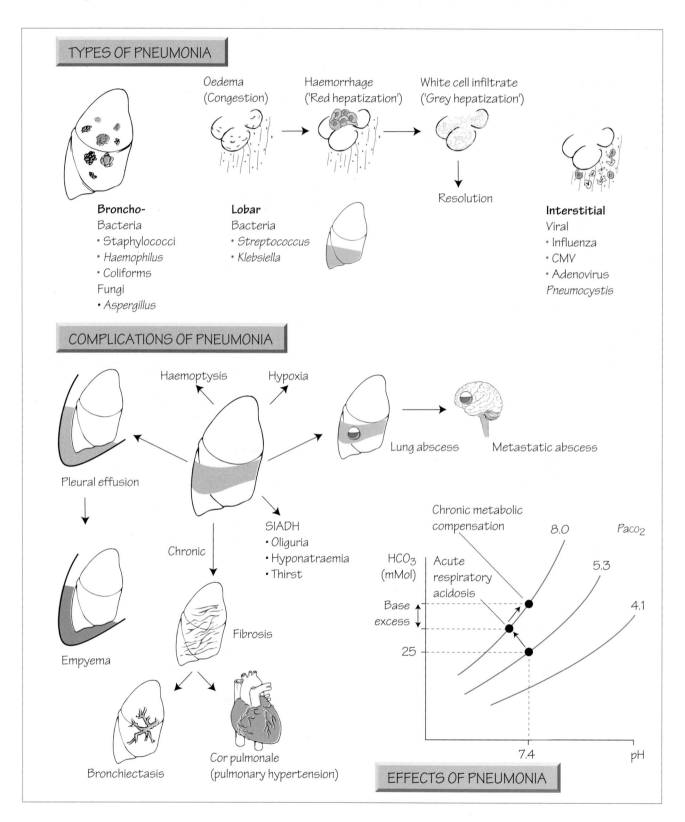

TYPES OF PNEUMONIA

Oedema (Congestion) → Haemorrhage ('Red hepatization') → White cell infiltrate ('Grey hepatization') → Resolution

Broncho-
Bacteria
- Staphylococci
- *Haemophilus*
- Coliforms
Fungi
- *Aspergillus*

Lobar
Bacteria
- *Streptococcus*
- *Klebsiella*

Interstitial
Viral
- Influenza
- CMV
- Adenovirus
Pneumocystis

COMPLICATIONS OF PNEUMONIA

Haemoptysis

Hypoxia

Lung abscess   Metastatic abscess

Pleural effusion

SIADH
- Oliguria
- Hyponatraemia
- Thirst

Chronic

Empyema

Fibrosis

Bronchiectasis

Cor pulmonale (pulmonary hypertension)

Chronic metabolic compensation

HCO_3 (mMol)

Acute respiratory acidosis

Base excess

25

8.0

5.3

4.1

$Paco_2$

7.4   pH

EFFECTS OF PNEUMONIA

Definitions

Pulmonary collapse or *atelectasis* results from alveolar hypoventilation such that the alveolar walls collapse and become de-aerated. *Pneumonia* is an infection with consolidation of the pulmonary parenchyma.

Key points

- Thoracoabdominal incisions are at high risk of postoperative pulmonary collapse and infection.
- Aggressive prophylaxis is key to prevention of complications.
- Postoperative pneumonia is often due to mixed organisms.

Aetiology/pathophysiology

Postoperatively patients frequently develop atelectasis, which may develop into a pneumonia.

Pulmonary collapse

- Proximal bronchial obstruction.
- Trapped alveolar air absorbed.
- Common in smokers.
- Common with chronic bronchitis.

Pneumonia

- Infection with microorganisms.
- Bacterial: *Streptococcus pneumoniae*, *Staphylococcus*, *Haemophilus influenzae*.
- Viral: influenza, CMV.
- Fungal: *Candida*, *Aspergillus*.
- Protozoal: *Pneumocystis*, *Toxoplasma*.

Predisposing factors

- Secretional airway obstruction.
- Bronchorrhoea postsurgery.
- Mucus plugs block bronchi.
- Impaired ciliary action.
- Postoperative pain prevents effective coughing (especially thoracotomy and upper laparotomies).
- Organic airway obstruction.
- Bronchial neoplasm.

Patients prone to severe pneumonia

- The elderly.
- Alcoholics.
- Chronic lung and heart disease.
- Debilitated patients.
- Diabetes.
- Post-CVA.
- Immunodeficiency states.
- Postsplenectomy.
- Atelectasis postsurgery.

Clinical features

Pulmonary collapse

- Pyrexia.
- Tachypnoea.
- Diminished air entry.
- Bronchial breathing.

Pneumonia

- Respiratory distress.
- Painful dyspnoea.
- Tachypnoea.
- Productive cough ± haemoptysis.
- Hypoxia—confusion.
- Diminished air entry.
- Consolidation.
- Pleural rub.
- Cyanosis.

Investigations

- Chest X-ray: consolidation, pleural effusion, interstitial infiltrates, air-fluid cysts.
- Sputum culture: essential for correct antibiotic treatment.
- Blood gas analysis: diagnosis of respiratory failure.

Essential management

Prophylaxis

- Preoperative deep-breathing exercises.
- Incentive spirometry.
- Adequate analgesia postoperatively.
- Early ambulation.

Treatment

- Intensive chest physiotherapy.
- Respiratory support: humidified O_2 therapy; adequate hydration; bronchodilators if bronchospasm is present.
- Specific antimicrobial therapy.

Complications

- Respiratory failure.
- Lung abscess.

73 Bronchial carcinoma

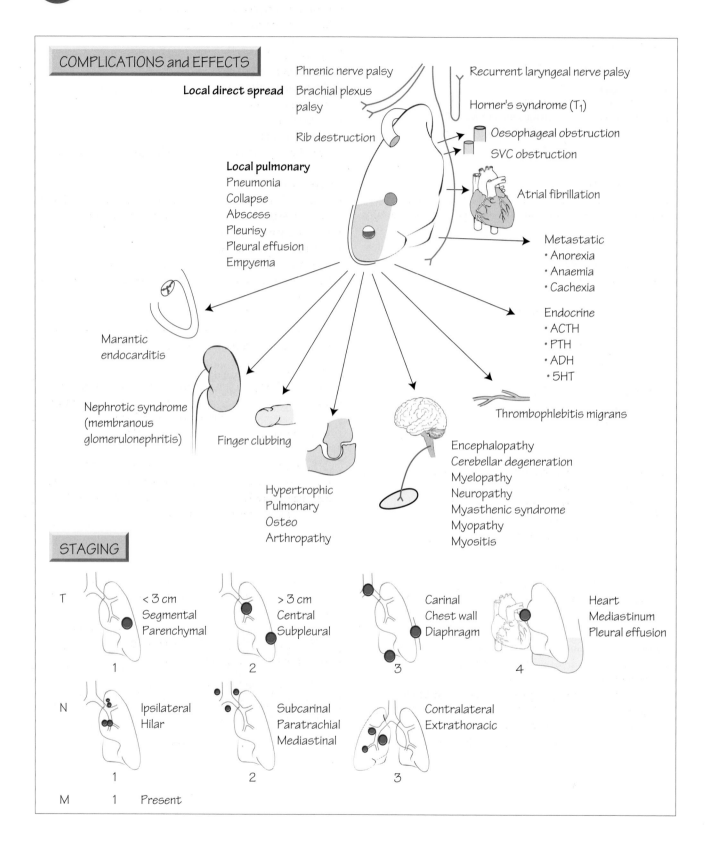

COMPLICATIONS and EFFECTS

Phrenic nerve palsy

Recurrent laryngeal nerve palsy

Local direct spread Brachial plexus palsy

Horner's syndrome (T_1)

Rib destruction

Oesophageal obstruction

SVC obstruction

Local pulmonary
Pneumonia
Collapse
Abscess
Pleurisy
Pleural effusion
Empyema

Atrial fibrillation

Metastatic
• Anorexia
• Anaemia
• Cachexia

Endocrine
• ACTH
• PTH
• ADH
• 5HT

Marantic endocarditis

Thrombophlebitis migrans

Nephrotic syndrome (membranous glomerulonephritis)

Finger clubbing

Encephalopathy
Cerebellar degeneration
Myelopathy
Neuropathy
Myasthenic syndrome
Myopathy
Myositis

Hypertrophic
Pulmonary
Osteo
Arthropathy

STAGING

T

< 3 cm Segmental Parenchymal	1
> 3 cm Central Subpleural	2
Carinal Chest wall Diaphragm	3
Heart Mediastinum Pleural effusion	4

N

Ipsilateral Hilar	1
Subcarinal Paratrachial Mediastinal	2
Contralateral Extrathoracic	3

M   1   Present

Definition

Malignant lesion of the respiratory tree epithelium.

Key points

- Symptoms may be masked by coexistent lung pathology (COPD).
- Bronchial carcinoma often presents late and most are non-resectable.
- Surgically resectable tumours have a fair prognosis.

Epidemiology

Male/female 5 : 1. Uncommon before 50 years. Most patients are in their 60s. Accounts for 40 000 deaths per annum in the UK.

Aetiology

The following are predisposing factors.

- Cigarette smoking.
- Air pollution.
- Exposure to uranium, chromium, arsenic, haematite and asbestos.

Pathology

Histology

- Squamous carcinoma: 50%.
- Small-cell (oat-cell) carcinoma: 35%.
- Adenocarcinoma: 15%.

Spread

- Direct to pleura, recurrent laryngeal nerve, pericardium, oesophagus, brachial plexus.
- Lymphatic to mediastinal and cervical nodes.
- Haematogenous to liver, bone, brain, adrenals.
- Transcoelomic pleural seedlings and effusion.

Clinical features

- History of tiredness, cough, anorexia, weight loss.
- Productive cough with purulent sputum.
- Haemoptysis.
- Finger clubbing.
- Bronchopneumonia (secondary infection of collapsed lung segment distal to malignant bronchial obstruction).
- Pleuritic pain.
- Neuropathy, myopathy, hypertrophic osteoarthropathy.
- Endocrine syndromes (ACTH is secreted by oat-cell tumours, parathormone is secreted by SCC—hypercalcaemia).
- Pancoast's tumour (apical tumour invading sympathetic trunk and brachial plexus)—Horner's syndrome, brachial neuralgia, paralysis of upper limb.
- Dysphagia and broncho-oesophageal fistula.
- Superior vena caval obstruction.

Investigations

Diagnostic

- Chest X-ray—PA and lateral (lung opacity, hilar lymphadenopathy).
- CT-guided lung biopsy.
- Sputum cytology.
- Bronchoscopy and cytology of brushings or lavage fluid.

Assess operability

- Helical CT scan of thorax/abdomen: involvement of adjacent structures, hepatic metastases, multiple primary lesions.
- Bone scan: metastases.
- Liver ultrasound: metastases.
- Mediastinoscopy: involvement of mediastinal nodes.
- Lung function test: likely patient tolerance of pulmonary resection.

Essential management

Surgical

- Indicated only for non-small cell tumours when tumour is confined to one lobe or lung, no evidence of secondary deposits, carina is tumour free on bronchoscopy.
- Operation: lobectomy or pneumonectomy.

Palliative

Radiotherapy (small-cell carcinoma most radiosensitive): stop haemoptysis, relieve bone pain from secondaries, relieve superior vena caval obstruction.

Prognosis

Following 'curative' resection 5-year survival rates are approximately 20–30%, but overall 5-year survival is only about 6%.

2 Week wait referral criteria for suspected lung cancer

- CXR suspicious for malignancy
- Persistent haemoptysis in smoker or ex-smoker > 40 years
- Signs of SVC obstruction
- Stridor

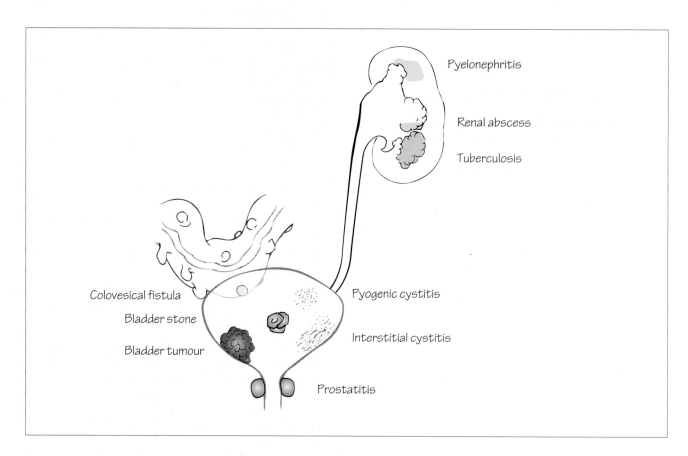

Pyelonephritis

Renal abscess

Tuberculosis

Colovesical fistula

Pyogenic cystitis

Bladder stone

Bladder tumour

Interstitial cystitis

Prostatitis

Definition

A *urinary tract infection* (UTI) is a documented episode of significant bacteriuria (i.e. an infection with a colony count of >100 000 single organisms per ml) which may affect the upper (*pyelonephritis, renal abscess*) or the lower (*cystitis*) urinary tract or both.

Key points

- Lower UTI is usually harmless and simple to treat.
- Upper UTI may be associated with renal damage and major complications and requires prompt investigation and treatment.
- Consider an underlying cause in all recurrent or atypical infections.

Epidemiology

UTI is a very common condition in general practice (usually *Escherichia coli*) and accounts for 40% of hospital-acquired (*nosocomial*) infections (often *Enterobacter* or *Klebsiella*).

Risk factors

- Urinary tract obstruction.
- Instrumentation of urinary tract (e.g. indwelling catheter).
- Dysfunctional (neuropathic) bladder.
- Immunosuppression.
- Diabetes mellitus.
- Structural abnormalities (e.g. vesicoureteric reflux).
- Pregnancy.

Pathology

- Ascending infection: most UTIs caused in this way (bacteria from GI tract colonize lower urinary tract).
- Haematogenous spread: infrequent cause of UTI (seen in i.v. drug users, bacterial endocarditis and TB).

Clinical features

Upper urinary tract infection

- Fever, rigors/chill.
- Flank pain.
- Malaise.
- Anorexia.
- Costovertebral angle and abdominal tenderness.

Lower urinary tract infection

- Dysuria.
- Frequency and urgency.
- Suprapubic pain.
- Haematuria.
- Scrotal pain (epididymo-orchitis) or perineal pain (prostatitis).

Investigations

Gram stain and culture of a 'clean-catch' urine specimen before antibiotics have been given. Usual organisms are *E. coli, Enterobacter, Klebsiella, Proteus* (suggests presence of urinary calculi).

Upper urinary tract infection

- FBC.
- U+E and serum creatinine: renal function.
- Renal ultrasound: swelling in pyelonephritis, stones, obstruction/hydronephrosis, secondary abscess.
- IVU: stones, structural abnormalities, obstructed collecting system.
- CT scan: abscess/tumours.
- Isotope scan (DPTA, DMSA): renal tubuloglomerular function.

Lower urinary tract infection

- FBC.
- Cystoscopy only if haematuria—underlying neoplasm or stones.
- If obstruction is present ultrasound scan, IVU and cystoscopy may be needed.

Essential management

Treat the infection with an appropriate antibiotic based on urine culture results and deal with any underlying cause (e.g. relieve obstruction). High fluid intake should be encouraged and potassium citrate may relieve dysuria.

Upper tract UTIs, epididymo-orchitis and prostatitis

- i.v. antibiotic therapy (ciprofloxacin, gentamicin, cefuroxime, co-trimoxazole).
- Relieve acute obstruction with internal (stent) or external (nephrostomy) drainage (especially if acute severe sepsis).
- An abscess will require drainage either radiologically or surgically.

Cystitis and uncomplicated lower UTI

- Oral antibiotics (trimethoprim, ciprofloxacin, nitrofurantoin, cephradine).
- If there is a poor response to treatment consider unusual urinary infections: tuberculosis (sterile pyuria), candiduria, schistosomiasis, *Chlamydia trachomatis, Neisseria gonorrhoeae.*
- Recurrent infections should raise the possibility of underlying abnormalities requiring investigation.

Complications

- Bacteraemia and septic shock.
- Renal, perinephric and metastatic abscesses.
- Renal damage and acute/chronic renal failure.
- Chronic and xanthogranulomatous pyelonephritis.

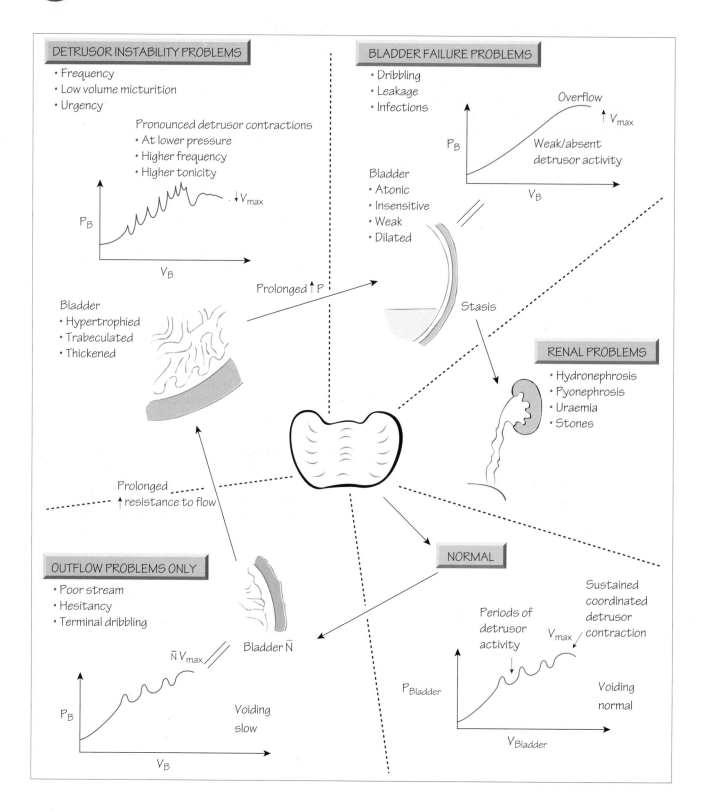

DETRUSOR INSTABILITY PROBLEMS
• Frequency
• Low volume micturition
• Urgency

Pronounced detrusor contractions
• At lower pressure
• Higher frequency
• Higher tonicity

P_B · $\downarrow V_{max}$ V_B

Bladder
• Hypertrophied
• Trabeculated
• Thickened

Prolonged $\uparrow$ P

BLADDER FAILURE PROBLEMS
• Dribbling
• Leakage
• Infections

Overflow
$\uparrow V_{max}$
P_B Weak/absent detrusor activity
V_B

Bladder
• Atonic
• Insensitive
• Weak
• Dilated

Stasis

RENAL PROBLEMS
• Hydronephrosis
• Pyonephrosis
• Uraemia
• Stones

Prolonged
$\uparrow$ resistance to flow

OUTFLOW PROBLEMS ONLY
• Poor stream
• Hesitancy
• Terminal dribbling

$\bar{N} V_{max}$
P_B
V_B
Bladder $\bar{N}$
Voiding slow

NORMAL

Sustained coordinated detrusor contraction

Periods of detrusor activity
V_{max}
$P_{Bladder}$
Voiding normal
$V_{Bladder}$

Definition

Benign prostatic hypertrophy (BPH) is a condition of unknown aetiology characterized by an increase in size of the inner zone (periurethral glands) of the prostate gland.

Key points

• Symptoms of BPH are initially due to outflow problems, then bladder instability, then bladder failure.
• Early treatment of symptoms prevents/reverses bladder damage and complications.
• Surgical resection is safe but is associated with some significant complications.

Epidemiology

Present in 50% of 60–90-year-old men.

Pathophysiology

• Microscopic stromal nodules develop around the periurethral glands.
• Glandular hyperplasia originates around these nodules.
• As the gland increases in size, it compresses the urethra, leading to urinary tract obstruction.

Clinical features

Initially outlet obstruction:
• Weak stream, hesitancy, intermittency, dribbling, straining to void, acute urinary retention.
Subsequent detrusor instability:
• Frequency, urgency, nocturia, dysuria, urge incontinence.
Finally detrusor failure and chronic retention:
• Palpable (or percussible) bladder, overflow incontinence.
• Enlarged smooth prostate on digital rectal examination.

Investigations

Basic investigations

• Urinalysis and urine culture for evidence of infection or haematuria.
• FBC: infection.
• U+E and serum creatinine: renal function.
• PSA: suspicion of underlying malignancy.

Further investigations

• Voiding diary.
• Uroflowmetry and residual volume measurement (normal < 100 ml): evidence of obstruction.
• Ultrasonography of kidneys and bladder: structural abnormalities.
• Transrectal ultrasound: to determine prostate size.
• IVU: structural abnormalities.
• Cystoscopy.

Essential management

Medical

• Alter oral fluid intake, reduce caffeine intake.
• α-Adrenergic blockers (e.g. phenoxybenzamine, prazosin).
• Anti-androgens acting selectively at prostatic cellular level (e.g. finasteride).
• Intermittent self-catheterization if detrusor failure.
• Balloon dilatation and stenting of prostate (unfit patient).

Surgical

• Majority of patients are treated surgically.
• Surgical removal of the adenomatous portion of the prostate.
• TURP with electrocautery or laser.
• Thermal ablation of prostate.
• Open prostatectomy if large which may be transvesical or retropubic.

Complications of surgical treatment

• Postoperative haemorrhage and clot retention.
• UTI.
• Retrograde ejaculation, impotence.
• TURP syndrome: in 2% of patients absorption of irrigation fluid via venous sinuses in the prostate causes hyponatraemia, hypotension and metabolic acidosis.
• Incontinence.
• Urethral stricture.

Prognosis

The majority of patients have a very good quality of life after prostatectomy (endoscopic or open).

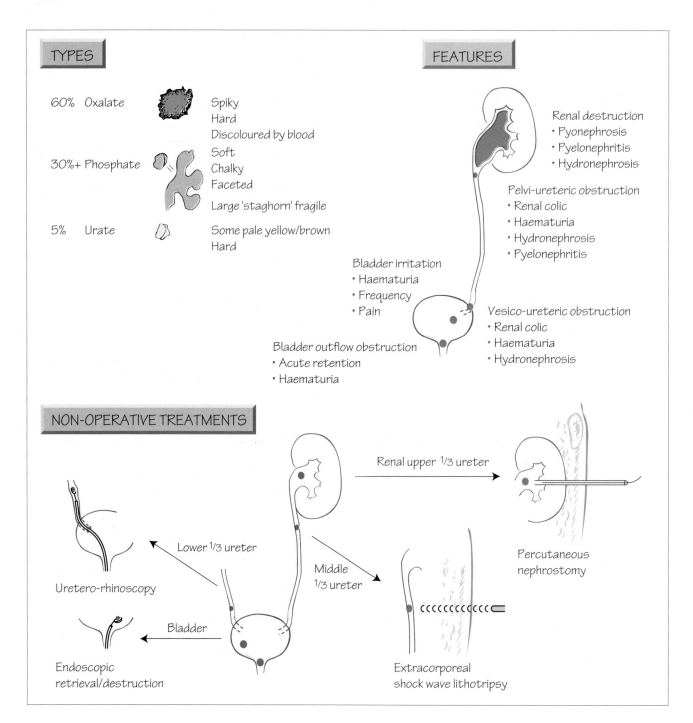

TYPES

60% Oxalate
Spiky
Hard
Discoloured by blood

30%+ Phosphate
Soft
Chalky
Faceted
Large 'staghorn' fragile

5% Urate
Some pale yellow/brown
Hard

FEATURES

Renal destruction
• Pyonephrosis
• Pyelonephritis
• Hydronephrosis

Pelvi-ureteric obstruction
• Renal colic
• Haematuria
• Hydronephrosis
• Pyelonephritis

Bladder irritation
• Haematuria
• Frequency
• Pain

Vesico-ureteric obstruction
• Renal colic
• Haematuria
• Hydronephrosis

Bladder outflow obstruction
• Acute retention
• Haematuria

NON-OPERATIVE TREATMENTS

Renal upper ¹/3 ureter

Percutaneous nephrostomy

Uretero-rhinoscopy

Lower ¹/3 ureter

Middle ¹/3 ureter

Bladder

Endoscopic retrieval/destruction

Extracorporeal shock wave lithotripsy

Definition

Renal calculi are concretions formed by precipitation of various urinary solutes in the urinary tract. They contain calcium oxalate (60%), phosphate as a mixture of calcium, ammonium and magnesium phosphate (triple phosphate stones are infective in origin) (30%), uric acid (5%) and cystine (1%).

Key points

- Calculi may develop because of or cause UTIs.
- Most stones pass without complication.
- Most stones are managed non-surgically.

Epidemiology

Male > female. Early adult life. Among Europeans prevalence is 3%.

Pathogenesis

- Hypercalciuria: 65% of patients have idiopathic hypercalciuria.
- Nucleation theory: a crystal or foreign body acts as a nucleus for crystallization of supersaturated urine.
- Stone matrix theory: a protein matrix secreted by renal tubular cells acts as a scaffold for crystallization of supersaturated urine.
- Reduced inhibition theory: reduced urinary levels of naturally occurring inhibitors of crystallization.
- Dehydration.
- Infection: staghorn triple phosphate calculi are formed by the action of urease-producing organisms (*Proteus*, *Klebsiella*), which produce ammonia and render the urine alkaline. Schistosomiasis predisposes to bladder calculi (and cancer).

Pathology

- Staghorn calculi are large, fill the renal pelvis and calices, and lead to recurring pyelonephritis and renal parenchymal damage.
- Other stones are smaller, ranging in size from a few millimetres to 1–2 cm. They cause problems by obstructing the urinary tract, usually the ureter. Calyceal stones may cause haematuria and bladder stones may cause infection. Chronic bladder stones predispose to the unusual squamous carcinoma of the bladder.

Clinical features

- Calyceal stones may be asymptomatic.
- Staghorn calculi present with loin pain and upper-tract UTI.
- Ureteric colic—severe colicky pain radiating from the loin to the groin and into the testes or labia associated with gross or microscopic haematuria.
- Bladder calculi present with sudden interruption of urinary stream, perineal pain and pain at the tip of the penis.

Investigations

- FBC, U+E, serum creatinine, calcium, phosphate, urate, proteins and alkaline phosphatase.
- Urine microscopy for haematuria and crystals.
- Urine culture: secondary infection.
- Plain abdominal X-ray: 90% of renal calculi are radio-opaque.
- IVU: confirms the presence and identifies the position of the stone in the genito-urinary tract.
- A renogram: may be indicated with staghorn calculi to assess renal function.
- 24-hour urine collection when patient is at home in normal environment.
- Stone analysis: origin.

Essential management

- Pain relief for ureteric colic: pethidine, diclofenac. High fluid intake.
- 80% of ureteric stones pass spontaneously. Stones of < 4 mm in diameter almost always pass, > 6 mm almost never pass.
- Indications for intervention:
  kidney stones: symptomatic, obstruction, staghorn;
  ureteric stones: failure to pass, large stone, obstruction, infection;
  bladder stones: all to prevent complications;
  sepsis super-added: nephrostomy.

Interventional procedures

- ESWL for small/medium kidney stones.
- Percutaneous nephrolithotomy for large kidney stones and staghorn calculi.
- ESWL or contact lithotrypsy for upper ureteric stones (above pelvic brim).
- Contact lithotrypsy or extraction with a Dormia basket for lower ureteric stones.
- Open surgery: ureterolithotomy or nephrolithotomy.
- Mechanical lithotrypsy or open surgery for bladder stones.

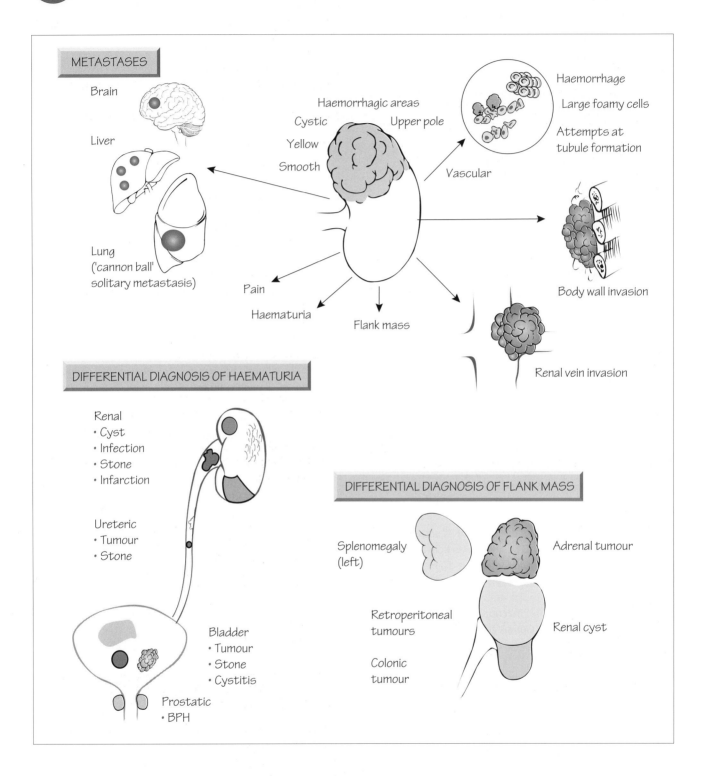

METASTASES

Brain

Liver

Lung
('cannon ball'
solitary metastasis)

Haemorrhagic areas
Cystic   Upper pole
Yellow
Smooth   Vascular

Haemorrhage

Large foamy cells

Attempts at
tubule formation

Body wall invasion

Renal vein invasion

Pain

Haematuria

Flank mass

DIFFERENTIAL DIAGNOSIS OF HAEMATURIA

Renal
• Cyst
• Infection
• Stone
• Infarction

Ureteric
• Tumour
• Stone

Bladder
• Tumour
• Stone
• Cystitis

Prostatic
• BPH

DIFFERENTIAL DIAGNOSIS OF FLANK MASS

Splenomegaly
(left)

Retroperitoneal
tumours

Colonic
tumour

Adrenal tumour

Renal cyst

Definition

Malignant lesion (*adenocarcinoma*) of the kidney epithelium (also known as *hypernephroma* and *Grawitz'tumour*).

Key points

- New, significant haematuria always requires investigation and may represent renal cell carcinoma (RCC).
- Consider RCC in unexplained anaemia, vague abdominal symptoms and recurrent UTIs.
- Surgery offers the best hope of long-term survival.
- Tumours are occasionally familial and a family history should be sought.

Epidemiology

Male/female 2 : 1. Uncommon before 40 years. Accounts for 2–3% of all tumours in adults and 85% of all renal tumours. (The other renal tumours are urothelial tumours, Wilms' tumour and sarcomas.)

Aetiology

Predisposing factors

- Diet: high intake of fat, oil and milk.
- Toxic agents: lead, cadmium, asbestos, petroleum by-products.
- Smoking.
- Genetic factors: oncogene on short arm of chromosome 3, HLA antigen BW-44 and DR-8.
- Other diseases: von Hippel–Lindau (VHL) syndrome, adult polycystic disease, renal dialysis patients.

Pathology

Histology

Adenocarcinoma (cell of origin is the proximal convoluted tubular cell).

Staging

- TNM staging.
- Robson stages I–IV
  Stage I: tumour confined within renal capsule.
  Stage II: tumour confined by Gerota's fascia.
  Stage III: tumour to renal vein or IVC, nodes or through Gerota's fascia.
  Stage IV: distant metastases or invasion of adjacent organs.

Spread

- Direct into renal vein and perirenal tissue.
- Lymphatic to periaortic and hilar nodes.
- Haematogenous to lung (large, 'cannon-ball' metastases), bones and contralateral kidney.

Clinical features

- Triad of haematuria (50–60%), flank pain (35–50%), palpable abdominal mass (25–45%). All three are present in < 10% of patients.
- Hypertension, polycythaemia (due to decreased blood flow to JGA → ↑renin, ↑erythropoietin).
- Anaemia, weight loss, PUO.
- Hypercalcaemia, ectopic hormone production (ACTH, ADH).
- Liver dysfunction (raised enzymes and prolonged PT) in the absence of metastatic disease.
- Renal carcinoma is one of the 'great mimics' of medicine.

Investigations

- FBC: anaemia, polycythaemia.
- ESR.
- U+E, creatinine: renal function.
- LFTs: metastases.
- Urine culture: infection.
- Abdominal ultrasound: assess renal mass and IVC.
- Helical CT scan: assess renal mass, fixity, nodes.
- IVU: image renal outline.
- Cavagram and echocardiogram: assess IVC and right atrium involvement.

Essential management

Surgical

- Offers best chance of long-term survival.
- Partial: if Stage I and part of VHL presentation.
- Radical: aim to remove kidney, renal vessels, upper ureter, adrenal and Gerota's fascia.
- Isolated lung metastases may also be removed surgically with good results.

Palliative

- Renal artery embolization (may stop haematuria).
- Chemotherapy (only 10% response rate).
- Hormone therapy (only 5% response rate).
- Immunotherapy (currently under review).

Prognosis

Overall survival is 40% at 5 years.

2 Week wait referral criteria for suspected urological cancer

- Macroscopic haematuria in adult
- Microscopic haematuria > 50 years
- Testicular body swelling
- Solid renal mass on imaging
- Increased PSA (if life expectancy > 10 years)
- Increased PSA with malignant feeling prostate / bone pain
- Suspected penile cancer

78 Carcinoma of the bladder

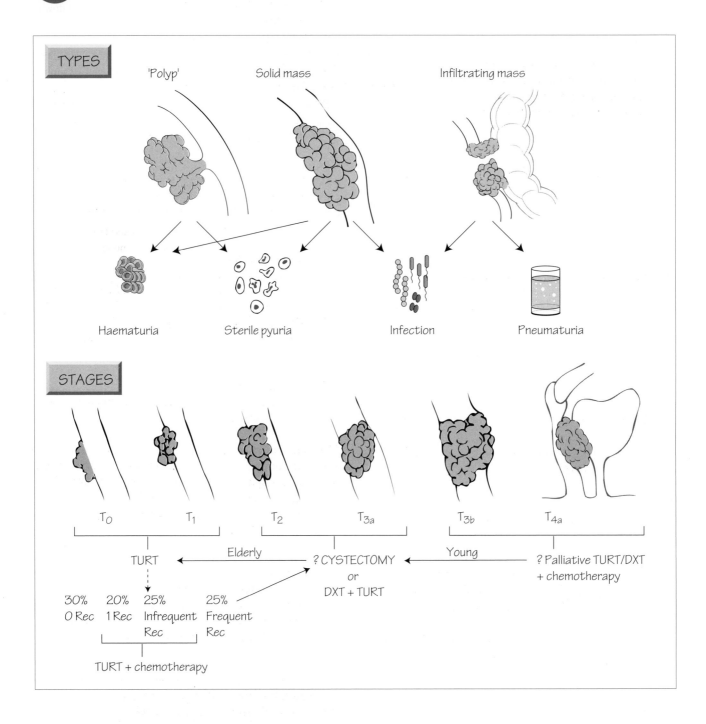

TYPES

'Polyp'   Solid mass   Infiltrating mass

Haematuria   Sterile pyuria   Infection   Pneumaturia

STAGES

T_0 T_1 T_2 T_{3a} T_{3b} T_{4a}

TURT ◄——— Elderly —— ? CYSTECTOMY ◄——— Young ——— ? Palliative TURT/DXT
                        or   + chemotherapy
                        DXT + TURT

30%   20%   25%   25%
0 Rec 1 Rec Infrequent Frequent
              Rec   Rec

TURT + chemotherapy

Definition
Malignant lesion of the bladder epithelium.

Key points

- Commonly presents with haematuria.
- Ranges from 'benign' acting recurrent bladder 'polyps' to rapidly progressive infiltrating masses.
- Transitional cell lesions are a 'field' change and often multiple.

Epidemiology
Male > female. Uncommon before 50 years. Increasing incidence of bladder cancer in recent years. Death rate is 7.6/100 000.

Aetiology
Predisposing factors:
- Exposure to carcinogens in rubber industry (1- and 2-naphthylamine, benzidine, aminobiphenyl).
- Smoking, tryptophan metabolites, phenacitan.
- Bladder schistosomiasis, and chronic bladder stones (squamous carcinoma).
- Congenital abnormalities (extrophy of the bladder) (adenocarcinoma).

Pathology
Histology
- Transitional cell carcinoma (TCC).
- Squamous cell carcinoma (rare).
- Adenocarcinoma (rare).

Staging for TCC

	T_{IS}	Carcinoma *in situ*
Superficial tumours	T_a	Tumour confined to urothelium
	T_1	Lamina propria involved
Invasive tumours	T_2	Superficial muscle invasion
	T_{3a}	Deep muscle invasion
	T_{3b}	Serosal involvement
Fixed tumours	T_{4a}	Invasion of prostate, uterus or vagina
	T_{4b}	Fixation to pelvic wall

Spread
- Direct into pelvic viscera (prostate, uterus, vagina, colon, rectum).
- Lymphatic to periaortic nodes.
- Haematogenous to liver and lung.

Clinical features
- Painless intermittent haematuria (95%).
- Dysuria or frequency (10%).

Investigations
- Urine cytology.
- IVU: occult upper tract tumours.
- Cystourethroscopy.
- FBC: anaemia.
- U+E creatinine: renal function.
- Ultrasound: obstruction.
- CT scan: local invasion, distant metastases.

Essential management

Carcinoma *in situ* (T_{IS})
- Intravesical chemotherapy for isolated carcinoma *in situ* and associated with papillary tumours.
- Cystourethrectomy for unresponsive lesions and 'malignant' cystitis.

Superficial tumours (T_a, T_1)
- TURT and follow-up cystoscopy.
- If recurrences or increased risk of invasion (large tumours, multiple tumours, severe dysplasia or carcinoma *in situ*) intravesical chemotherapy (mitomycin-C, BCG).
- Persistent recurrences despite therapy—cystourethrectomy.

Invasive tumours (T_2, T_3)
- TURT + radical radiotherapy; or
- Radical cystectomy (and reconstruction or urinary diversion, e.g. by ileal conduit).

Fixed tumours (T_4)
- Chemotherapy: MVAC (methotrexate, vinblastine, adriamycin, cisplatin), CMV (cisplatin, methotrexate, vinblastine), Cisca (cisplatin, cyclophosphamide, adriamycin).
- Radiotherapy and TURT for palliation.

Prognosis
- Superficial tumours: 75% 5-year survival.
- Invasive tumours: 10% 5-year survival.
- Fixed tumours and metastases: median survival 1 year.
- Long-term follow-up required for life.

2 Week wait referral criteria for suspected urological cancer

- Macroscopic haematuria in adult
- Microscopic haematuria > 50 years
- Testicular body swelling
- Solid renal mass on imaging
- Increased PSA (if life expectancy > 10 years)
- Increased PSA with malignant feeling prostate / bone pain
- Suspected penile cancer

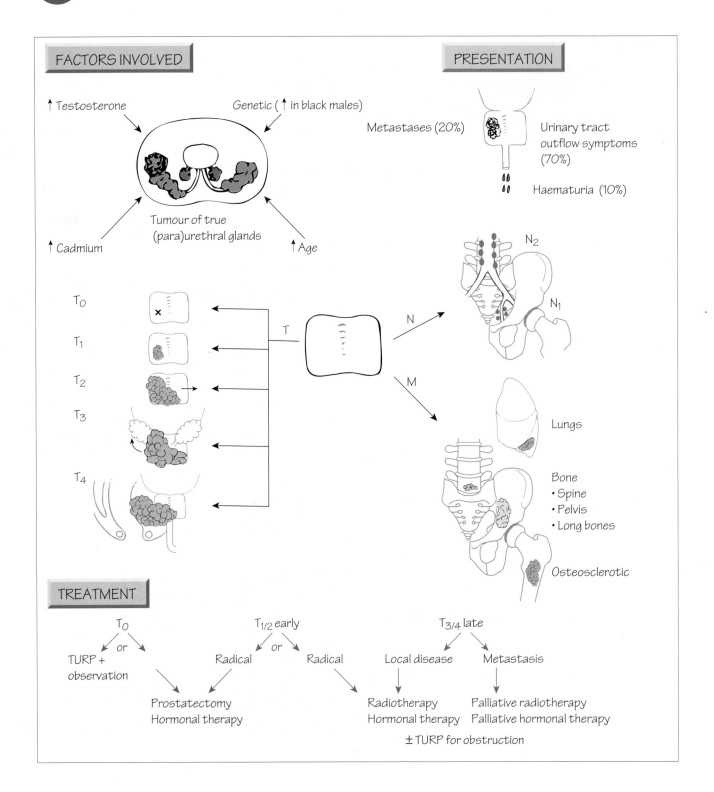

FACTORS INVOLVED

↑Testosterone   Genetic (↑in black males)

↑Cadmium

Tumour of true
(para)urethral glands

↑Age

PRESENTATION

Metastases (20%)

Urinary tract
outflow symptoms
(70%)

Haematuria (10%)

T_0

T_1

T_2

T_3

T_4

T

N

M

N_2

N_1

Lungs

Bone
• Spine
• Pelvis
• Long bones

Osteosclerotic

TREATMENT

T_0
or
TURP +
observation

$T_{1/2}$ early
or
Radical   Radical

$T_{3/4}$ late
Local disease   Metastasis

Prostatectomy
Hormonal therapy

Radiotherapy
Hormonal therapy

Palliative radiotherapy
Palliative hormonal therapy

± TURP for obstruction

Definition

Malignant lesion of the prostate gland.

Key points

• Prostatic cancer is common and should be considered in all new symptoms of lower urinary tract obstruction.
• Increasingly found (asymptomatic) by screening.
• Early treatment offers good 5-year survival with combined surgery and hormonal adjuvants.
• Late presentation disease is best managed medically and has a poor outlook.

Epidemiology

Uncommon before 60 years. 80% of prostate cancers are clinically undetected (latent carcinoma) and are only discovered on autopsy. The true incidence of this disease is considerably higher than the clinical experience would indicate.

Aetiology

• Increasing age.
• More common in black males.
• Hormonal factors: prostate cancer growth is enhanced by testosterone and inhibited by oestrogens or antiandrogens.

Pathology

Prostatic tumours are often multicentric and located in the periphery of the gland.

Histology

• Adenocarcinoma arising from glandular epithelium.
• Gleason grading (1–5) is used to grade differentiation.

Staging

	T_0	Unsuspected
Localized	T_1	Histological diagnosis only (clinical, radiology –ve)
	T_2	Palpable—confined within prostate
Local spread	T_3	Spread to seminal vesicles
	T_4	Spread to pelvic wall
	T_{1-4}, M_1	Metastatic disease

Spread

• Direct into remainder of gland and seminal vesicles.
• Lymphatic to iliac and periaortic nodes.
• Haematogenous to bone (usually osteosclerotic lesions), liver, lung.

Clinical features

• Bladder outflow obstruction (poor stream, hesitancy, nocturia).
• Symptoms of advanced disease (ureteric obstruction and hydronephrosis or bone pain from metastases, classically worse at night).
• Nodule or mass detected on rectal examination.

Investigations

• FBC: anaemia.
• U+E, creatinine: renal function.
• Specific markers: PSA, alkaline and acid phosphatase.
• Transrectal ultrasound and MRI: local staging.
• Needle biopsy of the prostate: tissue diagnosis.
• Bone scan: metastases.

Essential management

• T_0: observation, repeated digital (or ultrasound) examination and PSA.
• T_{1+2}: radical prostatectomy or radical radiotherapy, or interstitial radiation with ^{125}I or ^{198}Au.
• T_{3+4}: external beam radiation $\pm$ hormonal therapy.
• Metastatic: hormonal manipulation, bilateral orchidectomy, stilboestrol, LH-RH agonists, antiandrogens (cyproterone acetate), radiotherapy and strontium for bony metastases.

Prognosis

• Localized tumours: 80% 5-year survival.
• Local spread: 40% 5-year survival.
• Metastases: 20% 5-year survival.

2 Week wait referral criteria for suspected urological cancer

• Macroscopic haematuria in adult
• Microscopic haematuria > 50 years
• Testicular body swelling
• Solid renal mass on imaging
• Increased PSA (if life expectancy > 10 years)
• Increased PSA with malignant feeling prostate / bone pain
• Suspected penile cancer

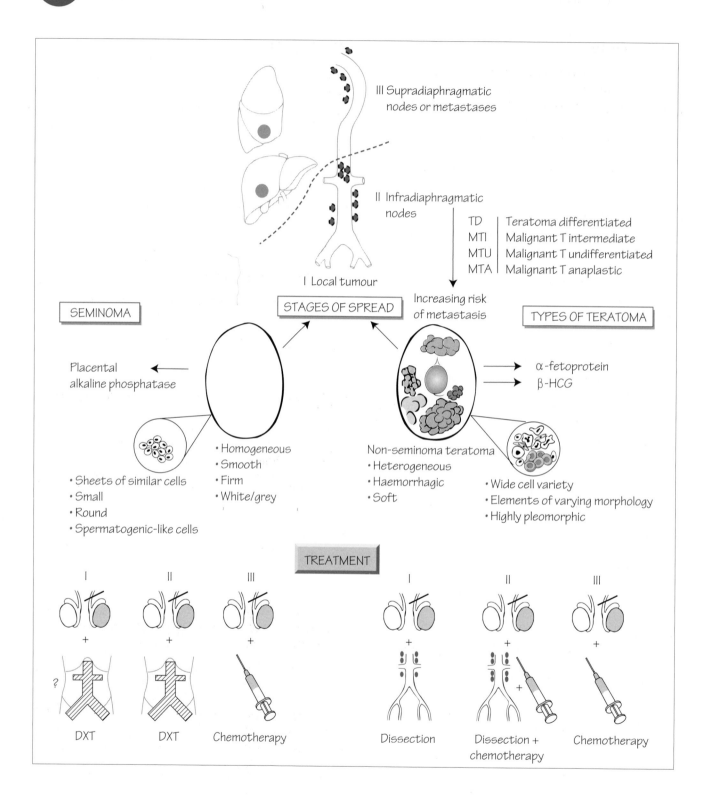

III Supradiaphragmatic nodes or metastases

II Infradiaphragmatic nodes

TD	Teratoma differentiated
MTI	Malignant T intermediate
MTU	Malignant T undifferentiated
MTA	Malignant T anaplastic

I Local tumour

STAGES OF SPREAD

Increasing risk of metastasis

SEMINOMA

TYPES OF TERATOMA

Placental alkaline phosphatase

α-fetoprotein

β-HCG

• Homogeneous
• Smooth
• Firm
• White/grey

Non-seminoma teratoma
• Heterogeneous
• Haemorrhagic
• Soft

• Sheets of similar cells
• Small
• Round
• Spermatogenic-like cells

• Wide cell variety
• Elements of varying morphology
• Highly pleomorphic

TREATMENT

I   II   III

DXT   DXT   Chemotherapy

I   II   III

Dissection   Dissection +   Chemotherapy
             chemotherapy

Definition

Malignant lesion of the testis.

Key points

- All newly discovered testicular lumps require investigation to exclude malignancy.
- Early tumours have an excellent prognosis with surgery alone.
- Late tumours have a good prognosis with surgery and medical therapy.
- Orchidectomy for tumour should be via a groin incision.

Epidemiology

Age 20–40 years. Most common solid tumours in young males.

Aetiology

- Crypto-orchidism—50-fold increase in risk of developing testicular cancer. Risk is unaffected by orchidopexy.
- Higher incidence in white men.

Pathology

Classification of testicular tumours

- Germ-cell tumours (90%) (secrete AFP and β-HCG):
  seminoma;
  non-seminoma—embryonal carcinoma, teratocarcinoma, choriocarcinoma.
- Stromal tumours:
  Leydig cell;
  Sertoli cell;
  granulosa cell.
- Metastatic tumours.

Staging

- Stage I: confined to scrotum.
- Stage II: spread to retroperitoneal lymph nodes below the diaphragm.
- Stage III: distant metastases.

Spread

- Germ-cell tumours metastasize to the para-aortic nodes, lung and brain.
- Stromal tumours rarely metastasize.

Clinical features

- Painless swelling of the testis, often discovered incidentally or after trauma.
- Vague testicular discomfort common, bleeding into tumour may mimic acute torsion.
- Rarely evidence of metastatic disease or gynaecomastia.
- Examination reveals a hard, irregular, non-tender testicular mass.

Investigations

- Blood for tumour markers, i.e. AFP and β-HCG.
- AFP is elevated in 75% of embryonal and 65% of teratocarcinoma.
- AFP is not elevated in pure seminoma or choriocarcinoma.
- β-HCG is elevated in 100% choriocarcinoma, 60% embryonal carcinoma, 60% teratocarcinoma and 10% pure seminoma.
- Scrotal ultrasound: diagnosis.
- Chest X-ray to assess lungs and mediastinum: metastases.
- CT scan of chest and abdomen: to detect lymph nodes.
- Laparoscopy (retroperitoneoscopy): to assess abdominal nodes.

Essential management

Radical orchidectomy (via groin incision) and histological diagnosis. Further treatment depends on histology and staging.

Seminoma

- Stage I: radiotherapy to abdominal nodes.
- Stage II: radiotherapy to abdominal nodes.
- Stage III: chemotherapy (bleomycin, etoposide, cisplatin).

Non-seminoma germ cell

- Stage I: Retroperitoneal lymph node dissection (RPLND).
- Stage II: chemotherapy + RPLND.
- Stage III: chemotherapy (+ RPLND if good response).

Prognosis

Overall cure rates are over 90% and node-negative disease has almost 100% 5-year survival.

2 Week wait referral criteria for suspected urological cancer

- Macroscopic haematuria in adult
- Microscopic haematuria > 50 years
- Testicular body swelling
- Solid renal mass on imaging
- Increased PSA (if life expectancy > 10 years)
- Increased PSA with malignant feeling prostate / bone pain
- Suspected penile cancer

Urinary incontinence

TYPES

STRESS
Pelvic floor injury

URGE
Detrusor instability

NEUROPATHIC
Head injury
Spinal injury
Peripheral nerve injury

ANATOMICAL
Vesicovaginal fistula

FEATURES

Volume infusion graphs

Pressure — Time
Leak
Cough

Pressure — Time
Detrusor contractions
Early voiding

Pressure — Time
Lack of coordinated reflex
Bladder reflex emptying

Pressure — Time
Normal curve
Dripping leak

TREATMENT

Ventral suspension
• Burch
• Stamey

Ant. vaginal repair

Anti-UTI
Vaginal oestrogens
Anticholinergics

Catheter
• Indwelling
• Intermittent

Repair

Definition
Urinary incontinence is defined as the involuntary loss of urine.

Key points

- A common and socially disabling condition.
- Full assessment and investigation is required to elicit precise cause and tailor treatment properly.
- Always assess if bladder full or empty (overflow or otherwise).

Physiology
Normal bladder capacity is 350–400 ml. As the bladder fills with urine, the detrusor muscle relaxes to accommodate the rise in volume without a rise in pressure (plasticity). When the bladder is full, stretch receptors in the bladder wall initiate a reflex contraction (via S3,4) of the detrusor muscle and relaxation of the urinary sphincter to empty the bladder. This spinal reflex is controlled by an inhibitory cortical mechanism, which allows conscious control over micturition. Conscious control develops during early childhood.

Classification
Urethral incontinence
- Urethral abnormalities: obesity, multiparity, difficult delivery, pelvic fractures, postprostatectomy.
- Bladder abnormalities: neuropathic or non-neuropathic detrusor abnormalities, infection, interstitial cystitis, bladder stones and tumours.
- Non-urinary abnormalities: impaired mobility or mental function.

Non-urethral incontinence
- Urinary fistula: vesicovaginal.
- Ureteral ectopia: ureter drains into urethra (usually a duplex ureter).

Pathophysiology
- *Stress incontinence*: urine leakage occurs when infra-abdominal pressure exceeds urethral pressure (e.g. coughing, straining or lifting), usually in the presence of urethral incompetence.
- *Urge incontinence*: idiopathic detrusor instability causes a rise in intravesical pressure and urine leakage.
- *Detrusor hyperreflexia*: loss of cortical control results in an uninhibited bladder with unstable detrusor contractions. The bladder fills, the sacral reflex is initiated and the bladder empties spontaneously.
- *Overflow incontinence*: damage to the efferent fibres of the sacral reflex causes bladder atonia. The bladder fills with urine and becomes grossly distended with constant dribbling of urine, e.g. chronic bladder distension from obstruction.

Clinical features
- Stress incontinence: loss of urine during coughing, straining, etc. These symptoms are quite specific for stress incontinence.
- Urge incontinence: inability to maintain urine continence in the presence of frequent and insistent urges to void.
- Nocturnal enuresis: 10% of 5-year-olds and 5% of 10-year-olds are incontinent during sleep. Bed wetting in older children is abnormal and may indicate the presence of an unstable bladder.
- Symptoms of urinary infection (frequency, dysuria, nocturia), obstruction (poor stream, dribbling), trauma (including surgery, e.g. abdominoperineal resection), fistula (continuous dribbling), neurological disease (sexual or bowel dysfunction) or systemic disease (e.g. diabetes) may point to an underlying cause.

Investigations
- Urine culture: to exclude infection.
- IVU: to assess upper tracts and obstruction or fistula.
- Urodynamics:
  uroflowmetry: measures flow rate;
  cystometry: demonstrates detrusor contractures;
  video cystometry: shows leakage of urine on straining in patients with stress incontinence;
  urethral pressure flowmetry: measures urethral and bladder pressure at rest and during voiding.
- Cystoscopy: if bladder stone or neoplasm is suspected.
- Vaginal speculum examination ± cystogram if vesicovaginal fistula suspected.

Essential management

Urge incontinence
- Medical treatment: modify fluid intake, avoid caffeine, treat any underlying cause (infection, tumour, stone); bladder training; anticholinergic/smooth muscle relaxants (oxybutinin, tolterdine).
- Surgical treatment: cystoscopy and bladder distension, augmentation cystoplasty.

Stress incontinence
- Medical treatment: pelvic floor exercises, oestrogens for atrophic vaginitis.
- Surgical treatment: retropubic or endoscopic urethropexy, vaginal repair, artificial sphincter.

Overflow incontinence
- If obstruction present: treat cause of obstruction, e.g. TURP.
- If no obstruction: short period of catheter drainage to allow detrusor muscle to recover from overstretching, then short course of detrusor muscle stimulants (bethanechol; distigmine). If all else fails, clean intermittent self-catheterization (neurogenic overflow incontinence).

Urinary fistula
Always requires surgical treatment.

Gastro-oesophageal reflux

Definition

This is a common condition characterized by incompetence of the lower oesophageal sphincter, resulting in retrograde passage of gastric contents into the oesophagus, leading to vomiting.

Aetiology

Immaturity of lower oesophageal sphincter; short intra-abdominal oesophagus.

Clinical features

• Vomiting, usually bile-stained, not related to feeds, may contain blood (indicates oesophagitis) and rarely is projectile.
• Failure to thrive may indicate repeated episodes of aspiration and pneumonia.

Investigations

If oesophagitis, stricture, anaemia or aspiration is suspected, a barium swallow, oesophagoscopy and biopsy, 24-hour pH monitoring and oesophageal manometry are indicated.

Treatment

• As there is a natural tendency towards spontaneous improvement with age, a conservative approach is adopted initially: thickening of feeds, positioning infant in 30° head-up prone position after feeds, antacids (e.g. Gaviscon®), drugs to increase gastric emptying and increase lower oesophageal sphincter tone (e.g. Cisapride®).
• Surgery (laparoscopic Nissen fundoplication) is reserved for failure for respond to conservative treatment with oesophageal stricture or severe pulmonary aspiration.

Infantile hypertrophic pyloric stenosis

Definition

This is a condition characterized by hypertrophy of the circular muscle of the gastric pylorus that obstructs gastric outflow.

Aetiology

The aetiology is unknown but it affects 1 : 450 children; 85% male, often firstborn; 20% have family history.

Clinical features

• Non-bile-stained, projectile vomiting (after feeds) beginning at 2–6 weeks.
• Baby is hungry, constipated and dehydrated. Loss of H^+ and Cl^- from stomach and K^+ from kidney causes hypochloraemic, hypokalaemic alkalosis.
• Palpable pyloric 'tumour' during a test feed or after vomiting.
• Gastric peristalsis may be seen. Ultrasound (or barium meal) if diagnosis is uncertain.

Management

• Correct dehydration and electrolyte imbalance with 0.45%
NaCl in dextrose 5% with added K^+. May take 24–48 hours to become normal.
• Ramstedt's pyloromyotomy via transverse RUQ or per umbilical incision. Normal feeding can commence within 24 hours.

Malrotation of the gut

Definition and aetiology

Malrotation describes a number of conditions that are caused by failure of the intestine to rotate into the correct anatomical position during embryological development. Midgut volvulus, internal herniae and duodenal and colonic obstruction may occur.

Clinical features

Bile-stained vomiting in the newborn period is the most common presentation but older children may present with recurrent abdominal pain, abdominal distension and vomiting.

Management

Surgery is required to release the obstructions.

Meckel's diverticulum

Definition

Meckel's diverticulum is the remnant of the vitello-intestinal duct forming a blind-ending pouch on the antimesenteric border of the terminal ileum and is present in 2% of the population.

Clinical features

Most are asymptomatic. May present with rectal bleeding, mimic appendicitis (Meckel's diverticulitis), be a lead point for intussusception or cause a volvulus. Ectopic gastric mucosa in a Meckel's diverticulum is responsible for GI bleeding and may be detected by technetium pertechnate scan in 70% of cases.

Management

Surgical excision, even if found incidentally.

Intussusception

Definitions

Intussusception is the invagination of one segment of bowel into an adjacent distal segment. The segment that invaginates is called the *intussusceptum* and the segment into which it invaginates the *intussuscepiens*. The tip of the intussusceptum is called the *apex* or *lead point*.

Aetiology

• 90% are idiopathic.
• Viral infection can lead to hyperplasia of Peyer's patches which become the apex of an intussusception.
• Other lead points include Meckel's diverticulum, a polyp or a duplication cyst.

Clinical features

• Most common cause of intestinal obstruction in infants 3–12 months. Males > females.

- Presents with pain (attacks of colicky pain every 15–20 min, lasting 2–3 min with screaming and drawing up of legs), pallor, vomiting and lethargy between attacks.
- Sausage-shaped mass in RUQ, empty RIF (sign de Dance).
- Passage of blood and mucus (redcurrant jelly stool).
- Tachycardia and dehydration.

Diagnosis

- Plain X-ray may show intestinal obstruction and sometimes the outline of the intussusception.
- Ultrasonography may help showing RUQ mass.
- Definite diagnosis by air or (less common) barium enema.

Management

- i.v. fluids to resuscitate infant (shock is frequent because of fluid sequesteration in the bowel).
- Air or barium reduction of intussusception if no peritonitis (75% of cases).
- Remainder require surgical reduction.

Inguinoscrotal conditions

Acute scrotum

Definition

The *acute scrotum* is a red, swollen, painful scrotum caused by torsion of the hydatid of Morgagni (60%), torsion of the testis (30%), epididimo-orchitis (10%) and idiopathic scrotal oedema (10%).

Management

- All cases of 'acute scrotum' should be explored.
- If true testicular torsion, treatment is bilateral orchidopexy (orchidectomy of affected testis if gangrenous).
- If torsion is hydatid of Morgagni, treatment is removal of hydatid on affected side only.

Inguinal hernia and hydrocele

Definitions and aetiology

During the seventh month of gestation the testis descends from the posterior abdominal wall into the scrotum through a peri- toneal diverticulum called the *processus vaginalis*, which oblit- erates just before birth.

An *inguinal hernia* in an infant is a swelling in the inguinal area due to failure of obliteration of the processus vaginalis, allowing bowel (rarely omentum) to descend within the hernial sac below the external inguinal ring.

A *hydrocele* is a collection of fluid around the testis that has trickled down from the peritoneal cavity via a narrow, but patent, processus vaginalis.

Diagnosis

- Diagnosis of a hydrocele is usually obvious: the scrotum con- tains fluid and transilluminates brilliantly.
- Diagnosis of a hernia may be entirely on the mother's given history or a lump may be obvious.
- Strangulation is a serious complication as it may compromise bowel and/or the blood supply to the testis.

Management

Both hernia and hydrocele should be treated by operation to obliterate the remaining processus vaginalis.

Undescended testis

Definitions and aetiology

A *congenital undescended testis* (UDT) is one that has not reached the bottom of the scrotum at 3 months post-term. A *retractile testis* is one that can be manipulated to the bottom of the scrotum. An *ectopic testis* is one that has strayed from the normal path of descent.

Diagnosis

Most UDTs are found at the superficial inguinal pouch and associated with hypoplastic hemiscrotum and inguinal hernia.

Management

- Treatment is by orchidopexy and should be performed at 6–12 months.
- UDTs are at increased risk of developing malignancy, even after orchidopexy and require long-term surveillance.

RENAL

Typical outcomes
1 yr graft survival 90%
5 yr graft survival 65%

- Typical indications
  - Diabetic nephropathy
  - Glomerulopathies
  - Renal cystic disease
  - Renal arterial disease
  - Metabolic diseases
- Technical notes
  - Donor sources (cadaveric, LRD, LURD)
  - Graft placed in iliac fossa
  - Blood supply from external iliac vessels
  - Ureter implanted into bladder
- Typical complications
  - Acute rejection
  - Chronic rejection
  - Urine leak ('urinoma')
  - Vascular thrombosis
  - Lymphatic leak ('lymphocoele')

CARDIAC

Typical outcomes
1 yr graft survival 80%
5 yr graft survival 65%

- Typical indications
  - Cardiomyopathies
  - Ischaemic heart disease
  - Congenital heart disease
- Technical notes
  - Donor sources (cadaveric)
  - Fully anatomical transplantation
- Typical complications
  - Acute rejection
  - Chronic rejection
  - Recurrent coronary artery disease

HEPATIC

Typical outcomes
1 yr graft survival 80%
5 yr graft survival 55%

- Typical indications
  - Alcoholic disease
  - Viral hepatitis
  - Toxin induced liver failure
  - Autoimmune hepatic/biliary diseases
  - Metabolic diseases
  - Congenital disorders
  - Budd–Chiari syndrome
- Technical notes
  - Donor sources (cadaveric, LRD, LURD)
  - May be part of a liver or complete liver
- Typical complications
  - Primary acute non-function
  - Bile leak
  - Recurrent coronary artery disease
  - Vascular thrombosis
  - Biliary stricture

PANCREATIC

Typical outcomes
1 yr graft survival 75%

- Typical indications
  - Diabetes
- Technical notes
  - Pancreas and duodenum implanted into iliac fossa
  - Often with simultaneous kindey transplant
- Typical complications
  - Pancreatitis
  - Acute rejection
  - Vascular thrombosis

SMALL BOWEL

Typical outcomes
1 yr graft survival 60%

- Typical indications
  - Short bowel due to resection/ vascular accident
  - Congenital atresia
- Typical complications
  - Acute rejection
  - GVHD

LUNG

Typical outcomes
1 yr graft survival 70%
5 yr graft survival 55%

- Typical indications
  - COPD
  - Cystic fibrosis
  - Fibrosing alveolitides
  - Pulmonary hypertension
- Technical notes
  - Donor sources (cadaveric, LURD('domino'))
  - May be part combined heart–lung, double lung or single lung
- Typical complications
  - Pulmonary infection

Definitions

• *Transplantation* is the removal of an organ or tissue from one organism and its surgical implantation into another organism to provide structure and/or function.
• A *Graft* is the organ or tissue transplanted.
  Allografting (also known as homografting) is transplantation between organisms of the same species (i.e. human to human)
  Xenografting is transplantation between organisms of different species (e.g. pig to human).
• Grafts may be placed in the same ('correct') anatomical location (*Orthotopic* transplantation) (e.g. heart transplant) or in a non-anatomical (*Heterotopic* transplantation) (e.g. kidney transplant).
• The graft comes from *a donor* and is implanted into *a recipient*.
• Donors may be *cadaveric* (usually brain stem death victims if human), *living related* LRD (family members sharing large genetic elements with the recipient) or *living unrelated* LURD (altruistic individuals donating one of a pair of organs).

Key points

• All but identical twin transplants require immuno-suppressions.
• Graft rejection can be hyperacute, acute or chronic.
• Long term immunosuppression causes diseases in its own right.
• Kidney, liver, heart and lung transplantation are well established with high success rates. Pancreatic and small bowel transplantation are being progressively developed.

Immunology of transplantation

• Pre-existing cell surface antigens (e.g. ABO and related blood groups) stimulate pre-existing humoral immunity in the form of antibodies. All grafts must be ABO matched or hyperacute rejection will occur.
• Class 1 MHC antigens (e.g. HLA-A, HLA-B, HLA-C) exist on nucleated cell surfaces and stimulate activation of recipient CD8+ve (cytotoxic) T lymphocytes. Optimizing Class 1 matching reduces the risk of acute rejection episodes.
• Class 2 MHC antigens (e.g. DR, DP, DQ) are found on cells such as macrophages, monocytes and B lymphocytes and stimulate CD4+ve (helper) T lymphocytes. Optimizing Class 2 matching reduces the risk of mixed humoral/cell-mediated rejection.

Graft rejection

• Hyperacute rejection—occurs shortly after graft enters host circulation. Caused by preformed antibody recognition of cell surface antigens and can be largely prevented by crossmatching between recipient serum and donor cells.
• Acute rejection—can occur at any time if the life of a graft but is most common in the first months after transplantation. Caused by cell-mediated immunity against HLA antigens. May be reduced or prevented by immunosuppression.
• Chronic rejection—occurs after months and years. Causes may be multifaoctorial including low grade cell-mediated attack due to HLA mismatching, chronic infection, underlying organ disease.

Immunosuppression

• All immunosuppressives result in non-specific suppression of the immune defence and increase the life time risk of infection and certain malignancies for the recipient.
• Typical infections under immunosuppression include; CMV, herpes groups viruses, *Pneumocystis*, *Candida*, *Aspergilla*, *Cryptococcus*.
• Typical malignancies under immunosuppression include; basal cell Ca skin, squamous Ca skin, B-cell lymphomas.

Drug group	Effect	Side-effects
Corticosteroids	Suppress all inflammatory elements of the immune respsonse	'Cushingoid' effects
Antiproliferatives (Methotrexate, Azathioprine, mycophenolate)	Prevent cell-mediated cell mitosis and amplification of response	Renal and hepatic dysfunction, marrow suppression
Calcineurin blockade (Cyclosporine, Tacrolimus)	Suppress T cells and rescue IL-2 release	Nephrotoxicity
Biological effectors (Antilymphocyte globulin, OKT3 Anti-CD3 Ab, Anti CD5 Ab)	Block specific parts of the immune responses	Fevers, nausea, vomiting, myalgia

Graft-versus-host disease

• Caused by donor immune cells present in the graft mounting immunological attack on recipient tissues.
• Causes skin, liver and lung inflammation.
• May be reduced by perfusing the graft thoroughly prior to implantation to 'wash-out' donor lymphocytes.

Index